The
Forgotten Body

The
Forgotten Body

A Way of Knowing
and Understanding Self

ELISSA COBB

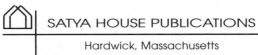
SATYA HOUSE PUBLICATIONS
Hardwick, Massachusetts

www.satyahouse.com

Printed in the United States of America

10 9 8 7 6 5 4 3 2 1

ISBN 978-0-9729191-4-2

Winter left when I wasn't looking.
It packed-up in the middle of the night,
And stole silently away
Like a secret lover who slips from the bed sheets at dawn,
Unheard, but somehow still felt.

It quietly lifted its icy fingers from my back,
Disappeared down the storm drain,
Melted into the tulip bed,
Evaporated in the March wind.

Just when I had resigned myself to its inevitability,
Accepted the need to wear the extra layers,
Stopped fighting with the woodpile,
And became accustomed to the daily chill,
Just when I stopped thinking "Winter,"
It slipped out leaving no forwarding address,
no thank you note, no business card.

Traces remain.
Deep puddles,
Soft smell of spring dirt,
Trickling streams down road shoulders,
Empty sleds resting on brown-green hillsides,
And that single glove that fell out of the car between
snow storms.

But somehow I yawned, gave in, fell asleep
And woke up to another season,
Wondering how I could have missed the departure
Of something I complained about so frequently.

And then I wondered about other things
That passed away like winter.
Parts of myself, old beliefs, stressors that I couldn't change,
Once accepted, once validated as my reality,
Also melted away,
Like turning around to speak to someone no longer
standing there,
Leaving only a trace of conversation hanging in the air.

Contents

Acknowledgements

This work is dedicated to my mother, Barbara L. Maranville, who had the hands of a nurse, the mind of a scholar and the heart of a warrior.

I also wish to acknowledge my husband, David, who loves, supports and encourages me in every way possible, my daughters, Jen Forest, Mary Christina Marion and Bridgette Spencer for the lessons they taught me through their growing up, my teachers and friends, Karen Kaumudi Hasskarl, Michael Lee, Peter Payne, Martin Prechtel, and Francis Charet, who touched my heart, allowed me to feel, and challenged me to stand in my own power, my spiritual sister Laurie Lowy for being an ever-present witness to my unfolding and a solid friend – no matter what, all of my many students, who are teachers in disguise, all those who generously contributed body stories to this work, Julie Murkette, for her editorial and publishing support and her belief in this book, and Carl Rogers for living and willingly teaching his faith in human beings to the rest of us.

Preface

One's body is an essential, yet often disregarded sage and teacher. Knowing and listening to one's body can enhance self-understanding and guide personal growth and change.

Through research, my personal experience of Yoga and Yoga Therapy, and the collected experiences of others, I have remembered that my body is a valuable source of transformational and affirmational information. In a culture where many have become accustomed to looking outside of themselves for guidance, this book offers the reader an opportunity to turn inside for the answers to questions about life and self.

I invite you to question what I have to say, while using your own experience as a lens of examination. Please take for yourself those aspects of my discussion that feel true for you. My work would be equally honored by both your agreements and your challenges to concepts that do not feel right. In the end, if I have provided you with a spark or two that can help light your way back to your own body — yourself — I will be pleased.

INTRODUCTION

The body is an instrument,
which only gives off music when it is used as a body.

— Anaïs Nin

The most profound pilgrimage I can ever make is within my own body.

— Saraha

Have you ever felt a low, consistent dissatisfaction with your relationship to yourself and the world around you? Well . . . me, too. And these feelings crescendoed as I entered my forties. The twists and turns of daily life, along with certain crisis opportunities, led me to more fully explore what psychologists might call "problems of the self." With an intellectual understanding of the body, as a twenty-year veteran of the fitness profession, I finished my Bachelor's Degree at Goddard College, focusing on mind-body studies — psychobiology. I entered the spiritual and physical practices of Yoga, Phoenix Rising Yoga Therapy (a healing modality that combines assisted physical postures and client-centered, non-directive therapeutic dialogue), and Qi Gong and rediscovered what I think I had always known: that my own body was my most reliable source of wisdom.

My years of experience with lifting the veil from personal authenticity through body-oriented practices such as Yoga have lead me to believe that present-moment *awareness of* and ongoing attention to one's body reveals vitally important information, insights and perhaps even revelations about self, relationship and purpose. The body — the process of being embodied — is an *essential*, yet often *forgotten*, source of knowledge and a key element of a successful transformative practice.

Having grown up in a world where, for the most part, the body had been viewed as a burden, problem, or even the root of evil, I have always had the sense that this way of looking at embodiment was somehow inappropriate. I have the same sense when I read yogic philosophy that refers to the body as the lowly or elementary aspect of consciousness and proposes body/mind transcendence. Instead, I believe that using my body's intelligence is a reliable, sophisticated way of knowing the Self, and it is well worth it to explore methods of translating the eloquent language of my body into day-by-day, useful information.

Yoga is a practice that integrates physical, devotional, intellectual and philosophical methodologies. It is a complex broad approach to the discovery and restoration of a human being's full potential in the light of one's relationship to Universal Consciousness.

Sri Aurobindo writes in *The Synthesis of Yoga*, "For contact of the human and individual consciousness with the divine is the very essence of Yoga. Yoga is the union of that which has become separated in the play of the universe with its own true self, origin and universality."

Yoga informs its practitioners about the aspects of Self through meditation, breath awareness, physical observation and 4000-year-old philosophical teachings. Transformation and the evolution of humanity, individual by individual, are at the heart of its purpose. In the practice of Yoga, change occurs through a deepening awareness of oneself in relation to all things.

There are many different forms of Yoga, each of which stresses one or more particular aspect of transformation. Some are more about embodiment, and others are more about transcending the limitations of the body. Overall, Yoga stands as a model for the developing union of psychology and spirituality. For thousands of years, Yoga psychology has *recognized* the critical role of the body in the quest for human meaning, authenticity and ultimately for the evolution of collective human potential.

As Yoga and its philosophies become integrated into Western culture, it is undergoing change that makes it applicable to responsible, contemporary life. And, in turn, Yoga is changing the face of contemporary life. Yoga, allopathic medicine, psychology and world religions such as Christianity and Judaism, are moving closer together, blending benefits. Western culture, in all of its diversity, has embraced many aspects of the philosophy and practice of Yoga — especially the physical ones.

My experience with Yoga as a transformative practice evolved from a growing compulsion to discover personal authenticity — the heart of my true nature, which was hiding behind a variety of mistaken identities. I was searching for proof of life — a deeper sense of self-meaning. My practice, which has been largely physical and philosophical, has slowly and clearly helped me to address "problems of self." Through establishing such a practice and integrating new awareness into daily experience, my abilities to self-mentor and self-soothe have evolved; a greater capacity for compassion has been attained.

My practice has evolved devotionally and intellectually. As it continues to do so, I find that I still consistently return to my body as the best source of guidance and information. It is through body awareness that I am able to contact the deep source of insight and wisdom that is universal in nature.

Each time I unfold another aspect of being, doing or knowing, I become more at ease with myself and my world of relationships. As I receive and integrate the information from my body (mental, emotional, sensory or spiritual), it reflects these shifts in consciousness through varying degrees of pain release, greater general wellness, posture improvements and decreased resistances to life flow. I continue to welcome it to reveal more of whom or what I believe is already at the heart of my being — a vastness, which is difficult to imagine much less to articulate.

While Yoga and Yoga Therapy have been at the heart of my transformative practice, I recognize that it is perhaps not best to not put all of one's eggs into one theoretical basket. As Mayan shaman Martin Prechtel once told me, "We need other things to save us from our orthodoxies." So my practice has also included journaling, creative writing, intensive retreats, Qi Gong, deep-tissue massage, dream work, reading/research, rites of passage study, solitary wilderness trekking and connection with nature. However, throughout this journey of self-revelation the mainstay of my practice has been and continues to be body awareness. Regardless of the chosen method or practice, the simple moment-by-moment experience of being embodied proves to be the most reliable way to knowledge.

I am not the only individual who, somewhere along the way, forgot how to be in my body. I have witnessed how reconnecting to body has flipped on the self-awareness-switch not only in myself, but also in others. By bringing one's relationship to body back into line with the intellectual, emotional and spiritual aspects of transformation, one's evolutionary journey truly begins. I hope that there are readers somewhere along parallel paths of discovery who might benefit from my shared knowledge and experience, as they create their own transformative practices. If not, then it may simply be enough to have had the experience of creating this body of work, knowing as scientific researcher Kurt Goldstein said, "Any change in one locality is accompanied by a change in other localities." If this is true, then in seeking and discovering one's own true nature, each individual contributes to the enhancement of the evolution of conscious, compassionate societies and cultures. This then speaks to the possible larger value of these theoretical offerings.

What Is Body?

When I say "body," I am referring to the exquisite, energetic network of cellular communication in which each sentient cell is fulfilling its life purpose on, within and beneath the permeable container we call "skin." Since our bodies provide us with tangible human identity and a direct experience of the surrounding world, it follows that they might also contribute valuable information in support of self-awareness and may act on our behalf as effective mechanisms of change. Within my own transformative practice of Yoga and Yoga Therapy I discovered an opportunity — an invitation — to reveal my authenticity. This invitation was enveloped in my learning of how to *focus on* and *translate* the language of the presently occurring phenomena and sensations of being a body.

The body is perceivable in a variety of ways both practical and metaphorical. Practically, our bodies allow us to negotiate and survive within both our physical and psychological environments. In addition it is now widely theorized in emerging science and psychology that memory, emotion and belief, along with life's joys and traumas, may somehow be stored in each of our highly intelligent cells and tissues and may be accessible — even reframeable through the exploration of sensation. Metaphorically then, our bodies, which have been with us throughout all of our experiences, tangibly integrate all aspects of Self and may well be our best and most reliable teachers.

My own body-informed, Yoga-based transformative practice led me to believe that my body cells and tissues *do* hold my story and also to more completely disregard the common notion that mind, body, emotion and spirit can be considered separately. As a library of the Self, the body allows us access to its metaphorical stories, though not all of its rooms are pleasant or comfortable, and not all of its books are initially translatable. I have learned that the study and integration process is simple, if not easy. Silence and attention are required if one is to be able to concentrate on the information stored in its many available volumes of truth.

Even during those times when our emotions are raw and we feel stripped of our usual defenses, when we cannot think any more, and we cannot find our spirit (the part of us that knows without thinking), we still have our physicality in whatever condition. All sensations are pregnant with the embryos of answers, waiting for us to surrender to self-awareness. I can always find the next step somewhere in my body.

In this *body* of work I explore and document my particular perspective of embodiment, clarify the relationship between body and transformation and emphasize the importance of body in integrating physical, emotional, intellectual and spiritual energies.

What Is an Authentic Transformative Practice?

True enough, change is as common and constant as the seasons of the year or the rise and fall of the tides. Change is how life is lived. But there is a certain type of change that we dress up as "transformation," and it expresses certain characteristics. These include:

- *Awareness* that some sensation or feeling needs unique attention.

- *Intention* to find out more – to give attention to growing awareness and the subtle fluctuations of sensation.

- *Willingness* to validate experience as *real, genuine and true.*

- *Action* or working through and deepening/clarifying aspects of awareness, exploring whatever arises from awareness and intentional attention.

- *Arriving* or internalizing/owning revealed self-discoveries, which then lead to a sense that one is genuinely different somehow, and noticing how that feels in the body.

- *Integrating* the new way of being with self and others into the flow of daily life and experiencing the body's way of acting as a guide.

An authentic, personal transformative practice is one that is characterized by these aspects of transformation and results in this type of integrated change.

Social/Cultural Context

At some point (or points) in life, the need or desire to define purpose, discover authenticity and find fulfillment moves into the foreground of our attention. We begin to question who we truly are and what we are meant to do. Healthy questioning regarding self, relationship and meaning, is often associated with periods of grief, fear, sadness, resistance, fatigue and pain. Perhaps our search begins with a gently growing sensation or discomfort similar to the pea under the princess's mattresses, or maybe we fall suddenly and unexpectedly into a transformational opportunity. However it begins, we end up not only in the search for our self but also for sources of knowledge and guidance – the metaphorical tools that will aid us on the path.

In our society there are tendencies to rely primarily on remedies from sources outside of ourselves, to label or to underestimate confusing discomforts and to fall into patterns of behavior that mask the reality of sensation. Even those among us who wish to actively claim responsibility for our own well-being often do not know how and where to begin. Caught in the rapid flow of personal and cultural expectations and demands, we find it difficult to turn and swim upstream in our effort to remember what I believe we were born knowing – our authentic identity.

As aspects of Yoga find their way into American life, contemporary psychotherapy appears to be evolving with an eye toward our larger community's (those who do not fall into the category of the mentally ill) hunger for the spiritual fulfillment offered by Eastern traditions. All disciplines seem to be moving toward a more holistic psychobiology of being, which includes aspects of psychology, spirituality, meaning and authentic awareness within (rather than transcending) aspects of daily human life. Remaining grounded in the human experience, while remembering our spiritual, divine nature is the unitary heart beating in the center of a new, expanding psycho-spiritual tradition.

Still, in mainstream America today it is difficult to support oneself through the inevitable twists and turns of self-discovery. While establishing a day-by-day transformative practice, it is easy to get lost in the gray area that lies somewhere between the valuable (yet not so easily accessible) contributions of Western psychology and the ancient wisdom of the yogis, which does not always readily fit into our "modern spiritual journeys." But we do always have our bodies! When I stopped overriding what my body was trying to say, when I stopped pushing the fast-forward button, I was amazed and grateful to discover what came up when I pushed "play."

Assumptions

- I am biased against what has become known as the body-mind split. Even though we are beginning to acknowledge that mind, memory and emotion are not actually separate from the body, but rather within the network of our cells, tissues and internal systems, we still speak as if we are disintegrated beings. I believe that mind, emotion, body and spirit are as inseparable as the components of our cells.

- The creation and establishment of an effective, transformative, spiritual practice can support individuals who have embarked on a path of self-discovery. The development of one's ability to access the body's wisdom through present-moment awareness of body sensations is an essential aspect of any successful transformative practice. To exclude or de-emphasize the body as a key source of evolutionary information is to separate oneself from a deep and reliable source of wisdom and opportunity for change.

- Although there are certainly times when consulting with allopathic professionals is of great value, no outer expert can know the truth about ourselves better than we do. We are our own experts when it comes to direct experience. Self-knowledge is a process that shifts into place through consistent moment-to-moment awareness of what is happening in the body. Psychologist Carl Rogers wrote, "Experience is, for me, the highest authority. The touchstone of validity is my own experience."

- Rogers added, "It is to experience that I must return again and again, to discover a closer approximation to truth as it is in the process of becoming in me. [. . .] My experience is not authoritative because it is infallible. It is the basis of authority because it can always be checked in new primary ways. In this its frequent error fallibility is always open to correction."

Here lies an opportunity for self-understanding, the possibility for clarity around life's issues and questions, and the potential for multi-level change and evolutionary paradigm shifts in consciousness.

Caveats

The realms of psychology, spirituality and personal story are full of jargon that can have multiple meanings for different readers. Words like "transformation" and "self" are imprecise and translatable in a variety of ways. In conversation we so easily speak of mind, body and spirit as separate entities that we hardly notice we are splitting ourselves apart. I have attempted to remain clear in my writing about what I mean by certain terms and concepts. I have also taken care to share with my readers the words of others accurately. I hope I have been successful.

I am standing on deliciously shifting ground. I hope that what I have to say comes across as *my* truth and not necessarily *the* truth. In the field of embodiment, mastery remains illusive.

Regardless of my religious convictions, political stance, skin color, racial heritage or sexual essence, *my* body tells the story of *me*. This, I believe, is true for us all. In addition, I am challenging beliefs about self that arise from these issues, such as self-desacralization and victim mentality.

Our personal stories, however, stand in the way of my basic point, which is that the body is an essential player in the process of transformation. After all, "The body is a very, very simple thing, very child-like, and it has that experience in such a compelling way, you know, it does not need to 'seek' anything: it's THERE. And it wonders why men never knew this from the start: 'Why, but why did they go after all sorts of things — religions, gods, and all those . . . sorts of things?' While it is so simple! So simple! It's so obvious for the body."

Two Cautions to the Reader

1. Once I remembered my body and learned to translate the language of self through the awareness of my cells and tissues, my body conversation has become never-ending. If this becomes true for you as well, you will always have to listen to that which you may not be listening to now.

2. There is nothing written here that you do not already know.

An Introduction to Yoga Therapy

Yoga is an ancient, multi-faceted, complex method of intense individual self-study that draws one's focus to one's whole-body, present-moment experience. It is a widely diverse tradition with many recognized varieties of physical and spiritual practices, all of which take root in the primary intention of Yoga — to accomplish a degree of union between the individual self and the vast totality of consciousness. Yoga Therapy, while strongly based on the philosophies and psychology of traditional Yoga, also offer the benefits of holistic techniques more familiar to Western sensibilities.

Yoga Therapy now falls under the wide-reaching umbrella of Yoga – a broad and complete system of understanding self and world. It is becoming a strong limb of the Western Yogic tree. There are two types, both of which provide support for growth and change. One is more physically therapeutic and prescriptive in nature. This type focuses on the anatomical and body alignment elements of Yoga postures in the presence of focused breathing. Its valuable emphasis is on physiology and the development of kinesthetic awareness in the practice of Yoga, as well as suggestions for living within the framework of a personally healthy lifestyle.

The second type is Phoenix Rising Yoga Therapy, a quite different, non-prescriptive, highly specialized, profoundly effective method of getting to know one's self through one's body. While also physically therapeutic, its approach is from a psycho-therapeutic direction. Throughout this book, the Yoga Therapy that I refer to is Phoenix Rising Yoga Therapy.

Phoenix Rising Yoga Therapy is a non-directive, client-centered, hands-on modality created by Michael Lee. During his own self-exploratory journey through Yoga at Kripalu Yoga Center in Lenox, Massachusetts, Lee completed his Masters thesis on the therapeutic value of Yoga. As part of this process, he began to experiment with assisted Yoga postures – stretches and poses in which one individual provides physical support for another with the intention of enhancing "what was naturally emerging from the body." In doing so, he witnessed himself and others making life-shifting discoveries. The ability to unravel the meanings of sensation seemed to be enhanced when postures could be visited with support.

From his experimentation, Lee eventually choreographed a rhythmic dance between the philosophies and beliefs of traditional Yoga and dialogue techniques reminiscent of the more holistic contemporary psychotherapies, particularly Carl Roger's theories of client-centered psychology and unconditional positive regard. The result is a "process for facilitating the client's awareness of what is happening in their body and their life, for integrating this information, and for using it to initiate desirable changes."

In Phoenix Rising Yoga Therapy, both client and practitioner co-create a session based on the intention and experience of the client. By visiting sensation in supported Yoga postures and positions, within meditative relaxation states, the client is able to become more deeply and honestly aware of his or herself. It is the focus of a Phoenix Rising Yoga Therapy practitioner to create and hold secure the external transformative space in which the client can safely explore the experience of being embodied, perhaps gaining "greater mental and emotional clarity around significant life issues, less tension in their bodies, and a more finely tuned awareness of their physical, emotional, and mental states."

A Phoenix Rising Yoga Therapy session generally consists of an opening, centering meditation in which to explore present emotions, thoughts and sensations, and sets an intention for what the client would like to receive.

The centering is followed by an exploration of body sensation and experience through certain client-indicated Yoga postures, stretches and other movements. Throughout the transitions from posture to posture, as well as in the stillness *between* transitions, an open-ended dialogue is included to invite a deeper experience of present self. The practitioner is trained to follow the client's experience rather than to lead it. Phoenix Rising Yoga Therapy maintains a very pure distinction between client-centered, non-directive therapy and clinical therapy, while using the domain of the body in therapeutic context.

Sessions conclude with a meditation of integration, during which the client has the opportunity to bring self-awareness into line with aspects of daily life.

No prior experience with Yoga is needed in order to receive the benefits of a Phoenix Rising Yoga Therapy session, nor does one's body need to be adept at movement. All that is required is a curiosity and willingness to explore one's way of being.

The benefits of Phoenix Rising Yoga Therapy are of value to a wide spectrum of clients. At one end of this spectrum are those who are seeking deep relaxation, while at the other end are individuals healing from highly traumatic life events. Phoenix Rising Yoga Therapy has been successfully used in conjunction with a wide variety of medical and psychotherapeutic modalities in the treatment of depression, illness, injury, substance abuse, addiction, chronic pain, stress related disorders and trauma related conditions arising from sexual and physical abuse. It has also proven effective for pre/post-natal support, smoking cessation, weight loss, family therapy, juvenile hyperactivity and special needs populations in school settings.

Since 1986, Phoenix Rising Yoga Therapy has proven to be appropriate and valuable to Western cultures. Lee writes, "As individuals become more technologically dependent and live more complex lives that require significant and frequent adjustments of focus and modes of being, they are more in need of a body-mind-spirit technology that can support them in making transitions with minimal stress."

There are over 1,000 Phoenix Rising Yoga Therapy practitioners in the world today, and close to 30% of those who seek certification are licensed, practicing psychotherapists who want to serve their clients in more effective ways. Others include physicians, medical practitioners, chiropractors, body workers and counselors, personal trainers and Yoga teachers.

My personal journey into Phoenix Rising Yoga Therapy, my intensive training to *become* a practitioner and my current work with clients has led me through doors of self-discovery that may not have otherwise opened. Phoenix Rising Yoga Therapy continues to enhance my own daily practice of traditional Yoga and likewise, my commitment to my daily practice enhances my ability to work as a practitioner of Phoenix Rising Yoga Therapy. The blend of Yoga and Yoga Therapy now form the widening lens through which I see myself and the world. This blend has become my chosen vehicle for transformation. This is how I am coming to know my true self.

PROLOGUE

It all started on the way to the movies,
followed by a very long walk in the woods.

July 1996 – Burlington, Vermont

"So what do you think?" I asked David as we pulled out into Route 7's pushy evening traffic.

Successfully negotiating a south-bound turn against the north-bound flow of rush hour, an act which seemed somehow metaphorical, he replied, "I think you should do it."

My body flushed with a few drops of adrenaline. "You do?" I wasn't sure if I was more surprised by his quick affirmation or by my own original suggestion.

"Yeah, I really do. I think it would be great! We've always talked about doing this. I'd love to go, too, but there's no way I could get away from work for that long. I'd really miss you, but let's talk about how you could work it out."

You know how people always say, "Be careful what you wish for." Well, this was one of those moments. I had somehow just made a decision to go for a 300-mile walk in the woods. What was I thinking?

The truth is that I was *feeling* as much as, if not more than, I was *thinking*. If you had asked me then, at the age of forty-three, why I wanted to do such a thing as hike Vermont's Long Trail from one end to the other, I would have answered, "I don't know. I just know that I'm supposed to. Call it a gut feeling."

I'm sure you know the kind of feeling I mean. It was a felt sense – a quickening – in my belly and other places. I don't remember the exact sensations, or just where in my body all these other places were. At that time I wasn't paying attention to such details. But I do remember that I was restless with overall *physical* urgency. There were parts of me that viewed this undertaking as a life-or-death, now-or-never proposition. Some clock was running. *Why* did not seem as important as *how* and *when*.

"I think that I really need to do this thing. I just feel a need to challenge myself. I can take a month off from work; August is slow anyway. They'll hardly know that I'm gone. I can borrow some equipment. I need to get new boots soon if I'm going to do this. And everybody says it's safe to go alone. I already know quite a few of the sections. I feel like its time to go – like if I don't do it now I might never do it." Within hours of the beginnings of those gut feelings, all this and more had come out of my mouth, almost as if someone else had spoken. It was with an almost surreal sense that I heard myself ask Dave that fateful question, "So, what do you think?"

My urgent "gut" feelings had risen up to the level of my throat, managing to escape as actual words. Now that my life-partner was encouraging me to transform these words into action, I knew that there was no turning back. The heat had just been turned up under whatever story-seasoned soup was simmering inside; the hike had already begun. Pride would have to overcome the immediate fear that smiled back at me from yet another inside place as soon as I heard David's response, "I think you should do it."

> *What is the way to the woods, how do you go there?*
> *By climbing up through the six days' field,*
> *Kept in all the body's years, the body's sorrow, weariness, and joy.*
> *By passing through the narrow gate on the far side of that field*
> *Where the pasture grass of the body's life gives way*
> *To the high, original standing of the trees.*
> *By coming into the shadow,*
> *the shadow of the grace of the straight way's ending,*
> *The shadow of the mercy of light.*
> — Wendell Berry

Looking back, my decision to take this hike was perfectly timed. I was just beginning to figure out some things about myself. Mostly, I needed to prove something to myself – something about ability and worth, about authenticity and purpose. I could see that I was my own missing link. I was never fully present to my life, and my absence was affecting my work and relationships.

A native Vermonter, I grew up on horseback in the little town of Bristol. My two sisters, who were much older, came of age and moved away from home before I was six-years-old, so I was an only child of sorts. An introvert who sometimes disguised myself as the opposite, I loved to draw, read, play guitar, go to school, climb trees, jump off the barn roof into the snow-covered horse manure pile and sleep in the stable curled-up in the embrace of my black Morgan mare.

At nineteen, I dropped out of college after my first year of art education study. My 4.0 average was not enough to fill the lonesome void I experienced from being isolated from my father who was dying of cancer. I was unaware at the time that I was creating my way home by allowing myself to get pregnant and married (an order of events that was embarrassing for my family). It worked. My first husband and I moved in with my parents, since we had no start-up money. Daddy died two weeks after the marriage ceremony. Our daughter, a blessing beyond words, arrived before I turned twenty. I had my marriage license before my driver's license, and I became a Mom while I was still growing up.

Seven years later, I was divorced and entering a second marriage to David and his two girls (now three daughters all together). I moved through jobs – house painting, retail buying and merchandising, paramedic, fitness professional, personal trainer and entrepreneur. Together Dave and I built and operated a health club in the early 1980s, well before so-called mind-body exercise was welcomed as part of the legitimate fitness scene. It turned out to be an exhausting twelve hours per day undertaking, but I loved the community that made it successful and considered the hard work well worth the effort. I was unaware of how the long, stressful hours were contributing to an impending crash.

Sudden turns in banking policies and market economy during the mid to late 1980s coincided with a breaking down of my self-defenses and opened up deep, raw, yet to be explored parts of myself. My fall into depression matched the fall of property value, and together they brought about the painful demise of our club. We lost a great deal of money, and almost lost our home and each other in the process. Sinking into what I can best describe as a black hole, I began Prozac and psychotherapy, while Dave and the kids looked on helplessly.

Why must the gate be narrow?
Because you cannot pass beyond it burdened.
To come into the woods you must leave behind the six days' world,
All of it, all of its plans and hopes.
You must come without weapon or tool, alone,
Expecting nothing, remembering nothing,
Into the ease of sight, the brotherhood of eye and leaf.
— Wendell Berry

At the bottom of this dark hole were family secrets about incest and the pain of these unspoken things. The very things that were supposed to go away simply because they had been avoided, had returned with a vengeance. I crashed into them, or they into me, afraid I might completely lose myself in the process. My body was sometimes numb – without sensation – other times clouded with unexplainable general pain. No one, myself included, really ever asked me about my physical experience of depression.

Therapy was difficult, and I dreaded every moment of it. I did, however, appreciate the warmth, understanding and skill of my therapist. She gently drew out many of the old roots that had been exposed inside my black hole and provided me with a flashlight so that I might find my way back up over its precarious edge.

My relationship both to my history and to my life situation softened as I gained clarity around family and events. The relatives that had needed to use my body in ugly ways had long since passed on; my father was one of them. My mother, who knew or at least suspected what had occurred, was alive but unavailable for comment on such things. I did quite a lot of intangible forgiving.

One particular therapy session marked a turning point in my healing process. During the hour, I released a significant amount of anger in a very physical manner – hitting pillows and yelling at the not present faces of my father and others. Although I was slow in getting started, initially feeling foolish, embarrassed and afraid of what might happen, I eventually allowed the dam of emotions to break. I screamed, punched, fought back, swore, wailed and cried for a good half-hour or more.

At the end of the session I was fatigued and somewhat bewildered, but also strangely able to be present to the strong sensations in my body as I walked out the office door to go home. I remember digging around in my tote bag with the feeling that I had forgotten something important. I even went back inside and glanced around the waiting room, sure that I had left something behind. Nothing found, I went back out to my car and realized on the way that what I had left behind was anger and blame. Maybe not all of it, but a heavy portion of my long-carried rage had stayed back there among my therapist's pillows. I was standing taller. My feet were lighter. Those who have long-distance backpacked probably remember what it feels like to remove a very heavy pack after a long day of hiking. I felt like that – like I could float away!

The freedom that I felt in my body that day was a turning point. The temporary feeling of floating transformed into a steady, more grounded one. I began to socialize, went back to caring for my family and started to work again. My energy slowly returned, my pain subsided and I remembered that I was capable of happiness. Years later I realized what had made that session so significant. *It was because my whole body had been involved.* My arms, legs, belly, heart and throat – every part of me – had participated in the process. Mind, emotion and the essential spirit that existed throughout me were expressed in a more holistic, integrated manner.

By 1996, I had stopped taking medication and had re-established myself as a personal fitness trainer and group exercise instructor. At this point in time, I did not have what might be considered my own physical or spiritual practice. However, I had taken advantage of

Vermont's many miles of scenic hiking, spending many days trekking with family and friends.

Vermont's Long Trail, affectionately known as "a footpath in the wilderness," is America's oldest long-distance hiking trail. Its more than 270 miles of rugged terrain meanders up and down the spine of the Green Mountains from its southernmost point near North Adams, Massachusetts, to the Canadian border near North Troy, Vermont. Traversing more than 100 mountains and heights of land, the trail offers sweeping views of the state's grand old valleys and villages, close encounters with wildlife and the promise of self-discovery. Each year a growing number of wilderness romantics and athletically driven diehards decide to take this daunting, yet doable, walk. I was no exception. So this evening in the Chevy van on an innocent Saturday night, drawn by the intrigue and magic of wilderness – in both nature's landscape and unwittingly in my own, I was proposing to hike this Long Trail from end to end, mostly by myself, beginning just two weeks from this movie date.

Thus, began the journey that catapulted me into an experience of body that years later, became the foundation for this book. It was on this walk in the woods that I began to remember that I was embodied wisdom. Silence, solitude and no escape from self made each step deeply meaningful. In the years that followed, my practice of Yoga and Yoga Therapy deepened my understanding of myself and of my body as an essential element of such understanding.

I did go on that hike, covering the distance in twenty-eight days. The following is an excerpt from my Long Trail journal entered on the last day.

The journey's end is not always what you think it will be. If it's not what you envisioned, you must look further and ask, 'Why not?' Do not become stuck here, un-ended. Keep trying to move, for you have changed in some way and that change must be explored no matter how afraid of it you are. A journey's end leads so quickly into the next journey that it is often cloaked from our eyes by the superficial layers of living. We cannot help but be temporarily submerged in the waters of daily life, but we must pull ourselves back to the surface now and again whenever it's important to look back at what was overlooked – to not move on so fast that we don't finish what we started. How will I finish this?

Gratefully, it did not "finish" at the Canadian border, nor has it ended yet. Sometimes when I close my eyes to sleep, I still see the image of my well-worn hiking boots moving along the trail. This journey of embodiment has turned out to be one of no return.

An Ongoing Conversation

The magic of my Long Trail journey was that I landed, slam-dunked, into a full experience of body. From the minute I first hoisted my fifty-pound pack into place, my body regularly spoke with me. Sometimes I listened, and sometimes I did not. When I didn't listen, the volume of my body's symphony increased. When I did listen, when I felt what was happening in my body and allowed myself to wonder about it, I experienced a wide spectrum of emotion and thought that included both grief and comfort.

In the rugged forests of Vermont many times there was no one to talk to other than my body. Often, the only sound was that of my own breath. It was difficult to avoid being with the thoughts, feelings and sensations that arose with relentless regularity. Sometimes the messages within my sensations were clear, such as when my shaking knees explained the advantages of taking slower, more focused steps – a technique I recognized as lacking in certain other areas of my life. And sometimes my body's attempts at conversation were clouded by my resistant un-readiness to fully explore certain aspects of myself.

I remember especially the deep, boney pain in my shoulder, which began about thirty miles south of the journey's end and eventually kept me from sleeping or eating. This discomfort was so great that for the final two days of my walk, I could function only when my pack was on, putting traction on the muscles and structures involved. Unable to escape the pain, I fought it with ibuprofen, afraid to fully experience its message, which in the end turned out to be, "Grieve."

So much accumulated grief from so many of my life experiences had risen to the surface of my awareness while out in the woods, but I still was not allowing its full expression. As I neared the end of the hike, my body urgently and desperately tried to persuade me to experience grief, and I still preferred the pain. It actually took two more years of chronic discomfort for me to finally allow my body to show me what it had been holding for years.

As I walked along the trail, I likened my body experiences to the metaphorical contents of my backpack. At those times when I realized that I had packed too much stuff – that my load was too heavy, I thought about the many things that I was carrying through life that no longer served me and limited my ability to move forward.

Later, when I began to consistently practice Yoga, I thought that what I was looking for was a new professional avenue. I intended to add Yoga to my tool chest of techniques with which to pique the interest of both my clients and myself. What I found instead through Yoga were those things that had remained in that pack, some of them ugly, some of them beautiful, all of them fascinating. The physical challenge of the postures, the stillness, the breathing, the patient listening to my body – all put me right back out on the long trail of my journey to discover my own true nature. My business-like intentions dissolved and, in their place my transformative practice matured.

Yoga means "to yoke" or "union." The ultimate intention of Yoga is to bring about the union of human and divine consciousness (the wider, universal energy which surrounds and resides in all things). Essentially, however, union or the lack of it can be observed in every moment of life, human or otherwise. Because we live in a dualistic world, we are provided daily with opportunities to understand and invite union. We can learn to see how two sides of one thing support each other, together creating a third thing, a middle perspective. By learning more about the characteristics of opposite things, we can paradoxically come to understand the deep connections between them. We can observe this both in the environment that surrounds us, as well as across the amazing inner landscape of body.

The body is an ever-present reminder of both duality and oneness. We consist of right and left sides, front and back sides, up and down sides, and inner and outer surfaces. We inhale and exhale and open and close our eyes, while our hearts give out and take in blood with each beat. We are living duality. And we are essentially one body — one whole human.

Regardless of the attention we choose to pay to the wisdom of body, body's wisdom remains present and accessible. Whether or not we eventually turn to the body as a source of vital information, the information is there. In my Long Trail journal on the last morning of my hike, I wrote:

> *The Long Trail is a microcosm of all that is. Not everyone is ready to see it so bluntly put. No arguments can be won out here against what is true. The trail magic is that it doesn't matter if you understand or not; it's just better if you do.*

What I was really writing about was my body. I could have just as easily written: "My body is a microcosm of all that is. Not everyone is (Am I?) ready to see it so bluntly put. No arguments can be won *in here* (in me) against what is true. The body's magic is that it doesn't matter if you understand or not; it's just better if you do."

Part One:

A Foundation

CHAPTER 1
BEGINNING THE FOUNDATION

We must assume our existence as broadly as we in any way can;
everything, even the unheard of, must be possible in it.
This is at bottom the only courage that is demanded of us:
to have courage for the most strange, the most inexplicable.
— Rainer Maria Rilke

The body is an important source of essential transformative information based on the following beliefs and assumptions:

- Cells are sentient (aware and intelligent).

- The network of our cells, tissues and body systems form both our practical structure for moving through our environment as separate and unique as well as hold the essential knowledge of our authentic nature.

- Cells have memory.

- What we commonly separate into mind, body, emotion and spirit are not at all separate. Though we are used to categorizing each of these aspects of self separately, they are really naturally overlapping and interchangeable experiences. What we experience as thought is actually sensation. Sensation can be felt as emotion, and our essence – our spirituality – may be discovered through our hearts or our bellies. Mind and emotion are not products of the brain alone; spirit is not separate from the body.

- Through our experience of being embodied, we are unique human focal points of one unifying consciousness.

- Authenticity – realness – is discovered through the process of revealing and remembering one's embodied divine essence.

- By paying attention to sensation and its corresponding emotions and thoughts, it is possible to find the answers to life's questions on the inside rather than relying primarily on external sources for such advice.

Exercise

Sit comfortably. Read the following short meditation and then either try it on your own, or ask another person to read it for you.

Close your eyes and imagine that there is a part of you that knows you without thinking about you – a part of you that is wise and loving toward yourself and always knows what is in your best interest. *(Pause)* Ask this part of you who you are and if answers come, do not allow anything to censor or edit them. If no answers come, simply keep imagining that they will come and be patient. Sometimes this takes a few tries. *(Pause)* If you find that you are unable to make sense of this exercise or the concept that such a part of you exists, then know that this is a real and valid experience in itself – not in any way a shortcoming. *(Pause)* What is it that you are experiencing as you consider this part of yourself? *(Pause)* When you feel complete with this exercise, open your eyes and write down the words that came out of this experience, whatever the experience was for you. Take as much time as you need.

Physiology and Anatomy –
A Matter of Depth Perception

It is highly dishonorable for a reasonable soul
to live in so divinely built a mansion
as the body she resides in,
altogether unacquainted with the exquisite structure of it.
— Robert Boyle (1627-1691)

Open just about any anatomy book and you will find beautifully drawn two-dimensional, colored representations of the body. These illustrations provide us with good frames of reference from which to learn the functional aspects of our anatomy. My point is this: most of us have grown up learning about the body from a two-dimensional perspective; we've seen it depicted horizontally and vertically on the pages of books.

As you read the following pages, I invite you to consider your own anatomy from two different perspectives: the perspective of actual sensation and the perception of depth. By actual sensation, I mean by simply noticing what is occurring in your body without evaluation, speculation or the need to change the experience. Depth perception perspective is also valuable when getting to know one's body. We are multi-dimensional beings in a multi-dimensional world.

Meditation

You may want a helper to read parts of this meditation to you.

In standing meditation (eyes closed), play with the possibilities of depth perception. Move through the suggestions that follow at your own pace. Begin by observing the space between the top of your head and the soles of your feet, allowing any sensations, thoughts, images and feelings to arise. Discover what is presently occurring inside your body between these two surfaces.

Next, let your focus shift to the space between the front and back surfaces of your body. Observe any information that stands out as interesting at the moment.

Now bring your awareness to the space between the right and left side surfaces of your body with the same exploratory attitude. Then turn your focus once again to what it is like to inhabit all of the space of your whole multi-dimensional body.

Turn your attention to the surface of your body – your skin. Notice which areas of it are the most familiar . . . and which are harder to become aware of. Notice the muscles beneath your skin, and any sensations or images that arise in association with your muscle tissue. Try to discover the deeper structures of your bones and joints. You might pick one and bring as much awareness to it as you can.

Another focus might be your heart, lungs or stomach. Ask yourself, "If this part of me could speak right now, what might it say?" With practice, it is even possible to bring a degree of awareness to other organs, such as kidneys, liver, and brain, as well as to the sensation of blood moving through arteries and veins. It is perhaps the easiest of all to notice your breath – its quality and quantity. Ask what your breath has to say about your state of being in this moment.

Through focused breath, turn your awareness, as much as possible, to the subtle flow of energy throughout your body. See what it is like to briefly touch upon the extremely subtle sensations of your body's perceptive systems (such as your nervous or hormonal systems).

Before you close such a meditation, locate the part of yourself that feels the most central to your existence at this moment . . . somewhere between your heart and your belly. Allow any flow of wisdom that is ready to come from this place. Then, in closing, turn your awareness back to the whole area that is your body – integrated . . . one body . . . right now.

When you are finished, you might want to write in your journal about your experiences. There is an element of continuation – a chapter-by-chapter flow of information – which you can go back and re-read, gaining greater clarity of self over time.

Consider yourself and other bodies in this multi-dimensional, depth perceptive, sensory sort of way. I hope it will make what I have to say simpler to understand and easier to integrate into your own philosophy.

The Sentience of Cells

> *Science says the body is a machine.*
> *The body says: 'I am a fiesta!'*
> — Eduardo Galeano

Human bodies are made up of approximately 75 trillion tiny units of life-energy called cells. These small rooms hold the information that make us uniquely human, create the energy that propels us through life and collect the data that result from our experience. Each one is both independent and also part of the larger community of cells that constitutes the network of all body systems.

For some reason, unknown by modern science, at a certain point in our fetal development our tiny hearts suddenly begin to beat. Yet even before this miracle occurs, the cells of our body already have mapped out the essential framework of our bodies and have created the tiny pump of a heart that will soon begin the thump-thump sound of "I am." And all of this intelligence occurs before our brain, the part of us that we consider to be the house of such intelligence, develops.

The more I learn about cells, the less alone and separate I feel. We are all comprised of trillions of microscopic aware beings resonating in communities of like-cells called tissues who consciously communicate on our behalf with other cells, tissues and organs across all of the systems of our functioning bodies. Each of our cells, with or without our direct input, is aware of its purpose in our body. Each constantly seeks environmental information and strategically adjusts itself accordingly.

In addition, the cells of *your* body resonate with the other cells in the bodies of those creatures that you come in contact with. Meeting another individual is a whole-body, all cell experience. For example, I recently met a person whom I had no logical or intellectual reason to mistrust, yet every cell in my body seemed to protest being near this individual. My body vibrated with alarm and confusion in this person's presence. I knew through my cells before I cognitively learned that my mistrust was well placed.

Moshe Feldenkrais defined intelligence as "the capacity to acquire capacity." In other words, intelligence is assigned to an entity that can change or develop its abilities according to its experiences. Our cells have such abilities and therefore can be said to be intelligent. Each has a known purpose, ability to communicate its state of affairs and "inherent self-righting tendencies" – the capacity to sustain its life and purpose through adversity and change.

At the center of my wonder about the sentience of cells – their capabilities to perceive and shift accordingly – is the mystery of why my first fetal heart cells decided to beat. From this wider perspective, the separateness that I have come to value as my individuality does not lose importance, but shifts into a place of deep connection. How could I really be alone?

These cells are the pearls of life.

— Yogi B.K.S. Iyengar

Dharma

In Yogic philosophy the term "dharma" is used to describe one's essential function or purpose for existence in this world. Cells have dharma, as do the tissues and organs that they comprise. For instance, the dharma of a bone cell is to resonate within a community of other bone cells to form bone tissue. One dharma of bone tissue is to provide connection and support. If the bone formed is a part of the spinal column, then its dharma has something to do with uprightness and mobility.

Another essential function of all cells and tissues is communication. This dharma is particularly noticeable in nerve cells and tissues whose life work is to receive, coordinate and transfer information about our environments both outside and inside our body. In association, the dharma of muscle tissue is to create mobility and stability and also to patiently wait for nervous system tissue to tell them whether to produce effort, hold tension or relax.

Cells and tissues also intelligently seek homeostasis. When things are out of balance, cells create ways to re-establish equilibrium so that all of the body's networking systems can continue to work on behalf of supporting life. Although this happens throughout the body in each cell, the endocrine and immune systems' tissues are great examples of this phenomenon. The dharma of endocrine tissues is regulation. For example, in relationship to our nervous tissues, they secrete the hormones that will help us mobilize for fight or flight when we are exposed to environmental danger. Later, they also produce the hormones that allow us to recover to our pre-danger, more relaxed state of awareness. In the case of our immune system, whose dharma is protection, cells are mobilized to seek and destroy foreign materials that can disrupt the balance of the body's systems.

There is growing evidence in support of cellular sentience and purpose through stem cell research and the controversial process of cloning. More is being discovered about the cell's ability to live outside of the body, isolated from other cells under certain controlled conditions. The cell appears to take with it all of the necessary intelligence to survive and even to multiply into new tissue communities. Continued perspectives into the lives of cells outside of the body may shed additional light on the process of cells in the body. Questions arise, however, as to the wisdom of separating parts (cells) from a whole (body) in order to understand the whole.

In possessing the dharma of relationship through community, connection and homeostasis, cells show us the physiological nature of their intelligence. The question remains: How far a leap is it to consider the possibility that each cell also contains the essence of consciousness – the "ultimate identity [dharma] of human beings."

The Amazing Network of Biochemical Potential

In it [the body] dwells the seers, the sages, all the stars and planets,
the sacred river crossings and pilgrimage centers,
and the deities of these centers.
— from the *Shiva-Samhit* (2.1-5)

The expanding world of neuroscience continues to discover and understand the biochemical substrates of thought and emotion as whole-body events. This, in combination with Eastern philosophical teachings, creates a broader perspective toward understanding the web of relationships that occur as a body. We develop what might be referred to as a sort of "ecological wisdom."

In particular, the work of researcher Candace Pert, author of *"Molecules of Emotion: The Science Behind Mind-Body Medicine"* provides a scientific perspective of the ongoing, ever-changing flow of self-informational energy that occurs in a body at any given moment. At the heart of her findings is this: The biochemical potential for thought, emotion, change and growth exists *throughout* the body via the universal, network-wide language of neuropeptides.

According to Pert, neuropeptides, the molecules of emotion, are strings of amino acids (protein-like substances), which regulate practically all life processes. They are produced in the tiny creative areas of cells otherwise known as the cell's ribosomes. Neuropeptides belong to a family of similar informational substances called ligands.

Keeping this in mind, consider one cell. Like all other body cells, its surface area is covered with millions of protein-based molecules called receptors. Each of these cell receptors has an opening that is something like a keyhole with long roots that wind their way deep down into the cell's interior.

Chemicals and other energetic charges, moving through the body outside of the cell, excite these receptors, causing them to vibrate and shape-shift between two or three favored shapes as they attempt to fulfill their purpose. They actually create a humming sound as they do this.

The receptor's job is threefold. Their first job is to scan the extra-cellular fluids for a closer look at the substances that have been exciting them, searching for the chemical key that will fit into their keyhole. The keys they are looking for are ligands which contain energetic messages for the cell. Depending on the type of cell, its receptors wait for just the right ligand to come along. This receptor specificity helps to ensure that the right messages get delivered to the right cell.

Once a key has been selected, the receptor's second job is to join with it, creating a union – a Yoga of sorts – between key and keyhole. Once inserted, the ligand creates a disturbance inside the receptor, causing it to fulfill its third purpose. The receptor rearranges its constitution so that the information from the ligand can enter the cell itself.

The chemical message that enters the cell via the ligand-receptor union causes the cell to change, sometimes dramatically. It affects the making of proteins, the opening and closing of various pathways of information, the addition and subtraction of certain chemical groups, and may also influence cell division – all of which can translate into changes in human behavior, activity and mood.

Neuropeptides, the molecules of emotion, are ligands. There are other ligands such as neurotransmitters (made by the brain and nervous systems) and steroids like testosterone and estrogen. But, neuropeptides (abbreviated as peptides) are by far our most prolific chemical keys, accounting for 95% of our body's available ligands. As with other ligands, peptides apparently affect our emotional state or mood. We could say that cells are the things that know who, how and what we are and, to some extent, they know what they know based on the choices our receptors make and the information contained within a specific peptide (or other kind of ligand).

Peptides prefer to move through the body via blood and cerebrospinal fluid, but they also can jump across the synapses (spaces) between our nerve endings. They easily travel the length and breadth of the body. Peptides and their partner ligands are the basic units of our in-body communication system, "by which our different biological systems interact and alter each others behavior."

The concept regarding this whole-systems phenomenon is illustrated by our immune cells, which make, secrete and store peptides that are the same as other mood-affecting chemicals produced by the cells of other tissues. In this way, our immune system can regulate our moods and emotions as effectively as our brain cells which can then reciprocally produce peptides that key into our immune system's cells. This exchange helps to clarify why emotional states are related to disease and the process of healing. Attitudes and beliefs can influence the onset of illness and vice-versa. For example, we are more apt to catch a common cold when we have a decreased amount of the happy state ligand, norepinephrine. In the absence of this hormone, empty receptors are more apt to make a union with a cold-causing virus. Once we are ill, our mood is influenced by our condition.

The ongoing dance between neuropeptides, ligands and cell receptors throughout the body unites our central nervous system (brain and spinal chord), peripheral nervous system, endocrine (hormonal) system, immune system, musculo-skeletal system, circulatory system, respiratory system and all remaining organs. (While considering the vastness of these systems' network, it is helpful to remember the multi-dimensional perspective mentioned earlier.)

The shifting, changing, overlapping exchange of energetic cues and responses moving in flows and waves across humming cell receptors may well be what we experience as emotion. Pert writes, "Peptides are the sheet music containing the notes, phrases and rhythms that allow the orchestra – your body – to play as an integrated entity. And the music that results is the tone or feeling that you experience subjectively as your emotions."

In this same way, Pert explains the concept of "mobile brain" – mind as "the flow of information as it moves [via peptides and specific receptors] among the cells, organs and systems of the body."

This network wide, multi-dimensional perspective of sensation, thought and emotion makes a good deal of sense. Emotion, which we experience as wave-like in nature, often seems to be more immediate than thought – accompanied by it, but not necessarily led by it. It has also been my experience that when I am aware, I notice that certain areas of my body respond faster and often more accurately to life circumstances than my brain does, although a certain unison of body thought follows. For instance, I may feel a sinking sensation in my belly or a squeezing in my upper back well before I receive a cognitive understanding of the particular situation at hand.

In fact, it appears that there is an unusually high density of neuropeptide receptors in the intestines, which might explain the sensations we describe as "gut feelings," such as the ones that led me out to the Long Trail. More recent findings by Wolfgang Prinz and Michael Gershorn reaffirm the nineteenth century theory of German neurologist Leopold Auerbach, and show that the digestive tract or "belly brain" has more nervous tissue cells than does our spinal chord. More cells and more receptors make this area rich in sensation, emotion, thought and essence. "Researchers believe that this belly brain may save information on physical reactions to mental processes and give out signals to influence later decisions. It may also be responsible in the creation of reactions such as joy and sadness." According to Prinz, this area of body "may be the source for unconscious decisions which the main brain later claims as conscious decisions of its own."

The same may be true for our hearts. An abundance of both peptide and neurotransmitter receptors on heart tissue (similar to those found on brain cells) indicate a chemical and neurological union between brain and heart and may explain why so much of our emotion is experienced in this place. Have you ever thought or expressed the words, "My heart knows . . . ." or "My heart is telling me . . . ?"

From his experience of working closely with heart transplant recipients, psychoneuroimmunologist Paul Pearsall has come to believe that the heart has its own intelligence and reacts to the world according to cellular memories (a concept discussed in more detail later in this chapter). It is not unusual for heart recipients to experience the memories and even the personalities of the donor.

In his book *The Heart's Code: Tapping the Wisdom and Power of Our Heart Energy*, Pearsall recounts several documented cases of memory traveling in heart tissue from donor to recipient. One case that stands out is that of an eight-year-old girl who received the heart of a ten-year-old girl who had been murdered and whose killer was still at large. During the recovery process, the younger recipient was able to accurately describe the events and details surrounding her donor's death, which led to the capture and conviction of the perpetrator.

Additionally, Paul Pearsall used Pert's findings to support what he calls the "continuous info-energetic relationship." Going back thousands of years, Pert's work shines new light on the Yogic concept of "prana," the life force that moves through all things and the Eastern concepts of "chi," the basic energy of life – both of which are said to be experienced as sensation.

All of this may help to explain why we experience emotion, thought and sensation as both somewhat different and also very much the same. They are linked and intertwined with each other. All are somehow tangible *and* illusive, material *and* immaterial.

Yet another thing we can "feel" through the music of this "orchestra" – this "body" – through the flow of peptides and the humming of receptors is *self*. Should Pert be on the right track, which I believe she is, then the amazing relationship she describes is literally the psychosomatic network of sensation, emotion, thought and, I suggest, *spirit* – essence of consciousness or self – which can be felt and known.

Now let's take another step down this new road of possible understanding. Because of their network of shared information/energy, each of the body's systems may have its own capacity for learning and memory (sentience). Hence, memory is stored not only in the brain cells via their receptor/ligand unions, but also at the receptor level of every type of cell.

In addition, Pert suggests that not only do peptides carry information, but they also cue cells and tissues to retrieve or repress information which was previously stored. She also notes that the quality and quantity of receptors that are willing to receive and integrate sensory and emotional information in both the brain and other body areas are apparently related to our intentions. We get a sense of the world around us, and, I believe, within us, "via our peptide/receptor rich way stations, each with its different emotional tone." The information that becomes conscious and that which remains unconsciously stored in our cells appears to be "mediated by our cell receptors."

Sensation, thought, emotion, memory, sentience, essence – such are the aspects of the interconnected flow of life information that is body. And it all begins at the level of the tiniest part of us – the cell. Or does it?

We can see how and where they seem to occur, but where do these aspects of our existence actually come from? If mind *is* this network, then what coordinates all of this? Is this embodied network the full extent of consciousness or a focal point of a universal consciousness that encompasses more than we can now imagine – or both?

These are important questions. While I love to wonder about them, I won't attempt to answer them. In fact, I'm not at all sure that I want an answer. What is to be gleaned from all of this, however, is whatever or whoever their ultimate source, body and mind are far from separate. From emotion to self-essence, we are inseparably and exquisitely one embodied energy.

On the last night of a four-day Yoga Therapy training experience I had a dream that left me with this image:

> *I have a cello, huge and beautiful with a secret heart.*
> *I need to unlock the secret of my heart in order to play the cello.*
> *I am not frantic to find the secret but curiously happy.*

The interrelated strings of the cello image reminded me of the dharma of networks. Because of its interconnecting nature, a network can be accessed from any point along its course of existence, and the entire network can be influenced from this point. If I place my hand on that secret cello place of my heart with the intention of clearly listening – sans censorship – to what is happening right there, right now, I can safely – without fear – enter into self-understanding, which turns out to be not so secret after all.

Cellular Memory

And there is always something there to remind me.
— Burt Bacharach (lyrics from *Do You Know the Way to San Jose*)

Memory as a Whole Body Event

Our life stories, stressful and otherwise, linger in our cells and body tissues. Each part of our body shares with our brain the responsibility of memory. It makes sense that something as important to our survival as memory would not be limited to a single organ storage area. Linked to learning, memory enables us to make choices and recognize the world around us. It is to our benefit to remember certain things, and sometimes it serves our purpose to forget. While there may be parts of the brain that help us with forgetting, there are other body tissues that take on the responsibility of holding those uncomfortable memories until we are ready to unfold the blessings disguised within them.

The concept of cellular memory is not a new one. Though never completely proven in scientific terms, many scientists and philosophers have believed it to exist. Ancient Yoga philosophy describes the existence of energetic cysts called samskaras. These cysts are believed to be stored past impressions from current and previous lives – neuromuscularly-encoded energy compressed or congealed within muscular and connective body tissues as well as within the general energetic field of the entire body.

Hans Selye suggested that experiences become "tissue memories" throughout the body because every part of the body is somehow "involved in the general stress reaction." Paul Pearsall adds his understanding of the stored "info-energy," which makes-up cellular memory, backing up his beliefs with the argument that "energy and information are the same thing."

How cellular memory might occur throughout the body is not fully understood. There is speculation about the involvement of certain cell structures in the memory process, such as cellular organelles. Each cell houses hundreds of these specialized structures, which appear to share an energetic/informational bond. Organelles, which perform specific metabolic (chemically reactive) functions, have memory of the energetic job they are supposed to do (their dharma). Other cell structures that may play a part in cellular memory are the microtubules. Microtubules form the lattice-like skeleton of the cell. They also perform as what can be thought of as the cells own nervous and circulatory systems of energy/information exchange. Anesthesiologist Stuart Hameroff has referred to microtubules as "a cell's own unique memory storage system." Pearsall writes, "It may be that cellular memories are not only neurochemical but also take place info-energetically at the level of the cell's microtubules."

The Gift of Stress

From my journal, August 2002, following Yoga practice:

Experience lands in my body,
Knots in my muscles, in my posture.
I am untying, unfolding
Knots or Nots?
Layers of knots untying
By honoring them as teachers, these protectors,
One thing cannot happen till another thing does.
Gaining simple freedom from fear and beliefs,
Tension safely dissipates.
It takes less energy to be untied.

Cellular memory and the stress of life go hand-in-hand. The events of life become embodied as they occur, and the effects of memory are likely related to the degree of stress surrounding such events. Hans Selye devoted a lifetime to pondering stress and its effects on living things. He wrote, "It is only in the heat of stress that individuals can be perfectly molded."

When I think back to the times in my life when I learned a great deal about myself, they usually paralleled or followed times of unusually great stress. However unpleasant, there always seemed to be something about the stressful situation that served to enhance my self-awareness and promote my evolution in some way. When I lost my fitness club business, I thought that I had lost myself and was in despair about my future. However, this experience of loss, in part, provided me with the time, opportunity and curiosity that eventually led me to the Long Trail. I might even go so far as to say the great loss and stress that accompanied it eventually led me to this book.

I know the stressful experiences of my life changed my self-perception and my outlook on the world. I also know my life experiences changed my body. Through my practice of Yoga and my increasing ability to notice my body, I became aware of my physical and emotional manifestations of stress – what Selye called "biological memories." For instance, I became increasingly aware of the bracing – the hardening of the musculature of my mid-back and of my tendency to protect my heart by slightly curving my shoulders forward. As I consistently explored how stress had landed in my body in a physical way, my posture, movement, and levels of peace and comfort have gradually improved. As I learned, through awareness, how I was in relation to my life, I was able to allow myself to be another way.

It has long been understood by holistic health pioneers and psychotherapists such as Wilhelm Reich, Alexander Lowen, Moshe Feldenkrais, Fritz Perls, Ron Kurtz, Ken Dykwald, James Gavin and others that our physical appearance – our postural presentations – are related to the ways in which we see ourselves in relationship to the world. Through our experience, our posture tends to become the objectively and subjectively observable representation of our self-beliefs and our expectations of those around us. Posture develops as body components become rearranged in relation to our assumptions, what Perls referred to as the "unaware manipulation of muscles," and Feldenkrais called "personal acture" or unintentional actions that prevent natural posture.

For example, if you assume that you will be attacked by life, you may either walk with a militaristic, forward-thrusted chest, braced for the inevitable blow, or you may slouch into a sway-backed position of defeat. While your posture has developed according to what seemed to serve you well, it may also impair or, at the least, limit your ability to move naturally and authentically. To move naturally and authentically is to move with effortless effort – fully aware of stress, but unattached to it.

The innocent beginnings of postural changes are sometimes rooted in what we might call fear-based tensions. While a certain amount of natural muscle tension is necessary to enable us to stand and move, fear-based tension refers to the continued holding-tight of muscle tissue when such muscle tension is not functionally needed. It is usually related to our sympathetic nervous systems autonomic response of fight or flight. For one reason or another, this system is aroused in preparation for some sort of danger, which may or may not actually be present. If the fight or flight never happens, the parasympathetic response of relaxation and return to homeostasis, which would normally follow a fully realized fight or flight, also does not occur. We remain stuck in expectation mode. Fear-based tension remains stored in the body tissues that were related to the experience which initiated the response to danger.

From my journal, August 2002:

The biggest risk I could take is to trust myself enough to trust Dave to come more fully into my life. Where do I feel mistrust in my body, when it seems directed towards me? In my solar plexus – right below my rib cage in the front of me – like knocking the wind out of my sails. It makes me really hurt, sad, then defensive, then hopeless, then I resign to it and keep the hurt inside because I understand where the mistrust comes from, and for a moment I think I must deserve it, although I have done nothing wrong. Then I close it in, retreat, protect, dissolve into pain there – the inmate on death row who is innocent and cannot prove it. I must remember not to dissolve myself into this part of our union, which otherwise feels strong. I have spent my whole life proving my innocence.

Another way that cellular memory can be appreciated is by reflecting on the many ways in which our bodies carry out their dharma without our conscious command. From our first spontaneous heart beat until our last, our bodies carry out functions that for most of us remain below the level of our daily awareness. Our blood vessels dilate and constrict to heat and cool us, our intestines move food and waste through great distances and our immune system destroys the interlopers who challenge our health. Over time, through repeated experience, our body evolves to act on our behalf without our thinking about it.

Exercise

Sit or stand with one arm extended straight out in front of you, your palm facing up. Then turn the palm down. Repeat this a few times. Chances are that when your palm is facing up, your fingers curve slightly toward the ceiling, and when your palm is down, your fingers tend to straighten out. There is no physiological reason for this to happen. You can easily change this through your awareness if you want to. However, your body – your hand – remembers that when your palm is facing up, it is likely that something will land on it and your fingers will need to be ready to close around whatever that thing is. And your cells and tissues know that when your palm is down, you are more likely to be preparing to pick something up, and your fingers spread open in readiness to do so.

If we believe evolutionist theories, then we must assume that our cells changed in response to our environment in order to survive and that a certain amount of memory about what worked and what did not work had to have occurred. Here, some pretty big questions arise. How is it that we are still in existence if certain of our species died due to such experiences – all that particular individual's memory supposedly gone? Did cellular memory travel in DNA from one individual to the next, or did consciousness itself evolve and reappear in a new individual form? Indeed, we can no more easily explain the existence and intentions of DNA than we can explain that first tiny heart beat.

Morphic Resonance Theory Explored

Contemporary researcher, Rupert Sheldrake, offers another view. He proposes that "growing organisms are shaped by fields . . . which contain, as it were, the form of the organism." Each field is "an invisible organizing structure which organizes [an organism's] development" and has "a kind of in-built memory derived from previous forms of a similar kind." According to Sheldrake the process of "morphic resonance" occurs within such fields – a process which connects one field to other similar fields. He suggests that the "field's structure has a cumulative memory, based on what has happened to the species in the past," and that this phenomenon applies across the spectrum of existence from living organisms to single atoms. Memory would then occur in the fields themselves rather than in our individual brains; the brain/body is viewed as "more like a tuning system than a memory storage device." Along these same lines, heredity is seen not only as related to our DNA, but also dependent on morphic resonance. We tune in not only to our own individual memories but also to the memories of others – a collective memory not unlike Jung's collective unconscious.

Initially it appears as though Sheldrake's views suggest that memory is not an attribute of cells, but rather of morphic fields. Yet, according to his views of the broad nature of such fields, it could be argued that cells might have their own morphic resonance, sentience *and* individual memory.

Bodies and Culture

Another version of cellular memory is related to culture and society. The term cultural comportment refers to the ways in which we hold and move in relation to the space around us, given the cultural norms and expectations imposed upon us. For instance, when performing movement aspects of daily living, Western women tend to have a more limited range of motion than Western men. Even though they may be more flexible (on many levels), women do not usually make use of their full potential range of motion in certain life movements such as walking. In regular walking, a woman's stride is shorter than a man's, and the arc of her arm swing is less wide even when her body is similar in proportion to that of a man's. Western women also tend to sit with their legs crossed and stand with their arms folded across their bodies. Without thinking about it, schoolgirls tend to carry their books in front of their chests, while boys tend to carry their books in one arm at their sides.

In addition, our bodies may be, to some extent, formed by our feelings of failure when we cannot comply with the consumer culture's unachievable expectations of the body to be perfect – young, slender, healthy, happy, well-exercised, sexy and capable of anything at any time. The Western consumer view of the body as a business appears to be losing no ground and, in fact, may be infiltrating into other cultures.

Cellular memory is not always old. Bodies may know wear and tear, but they do not know time as far as past, present and future. The life events that are occurring right now are already registering in our bodies. If we pay attention, moment-by-moment, we can gain valuable and immediate insight about what is currently happening to us, as well as what may have happened in the past and what might happen in the future.

What a Wonderful World!

Within this fathomlong body is found all the teachings,
is found suffering, the cause of suffering, and the end of suffering.
— Buddha

The Kingdom of God is within you.

— Jesus

Heredity, activity, exposure to and responses to the experiences of life, un-expressed emotion, thoughts and fears, cultural expectations, environmental stresses, beliefs about self and others – all of these things contribute to the memory banks of our body's cells and tissues. Ken Dychtwald writes, "The body begins to form around the feelings that animate it, and the feelings, in turn, become habituated and trapped within the body tissue, itself."

At the risk of asking you to take a leap of faith, I invite you to consider how wonderful all this is! Information about cellular memory tends to carry the overtones of a doomsday scenario for the human condition. *"Life experiences trapped in our body cells? Oh no! How bad is that? Memories are in there and will be there forever! It's just more that I'll have to bear and suffer through. And by the way it must have all been my fault somehow."* Not so!

Hooray for cellular memory! Thank goodness it exists. It is the key to our self-understanding and to our ability to reveal our authenticity. Yes, it may sometimes be painful to slowly weed through the things that have come to rest within us, but as we pull them out and understand their roots, we begin to be able to recognize the garden that was there all along, overgrown and forgotten. Part of the human experience is to get weedy. We cannot experience ourselves as human without the weeds. We cannot experience our divine true nature without first experiencing the contrast between the weedy garden and the well tended one.

Weeds, cellular memories, samskaras are interesting things. They can be pulled out, extracted or remembered only after they have first been welcomed and thanked for the worthwhile purposes they served. They are not to be yanked out prematurely, covered up or chased away, but rather they need to be offered an honorable discharge full of recognition and ceremony – perhaps even ritual. But even before that, cellular memories and the sensations, emotions and thoughts that are part of their entourage need to have time on center stage to tell their long-held story – to complete their dharma. Fritz Perls wrote, "The muscular tensions which prevent relaxation constitute important parts of the very resistances that we want to attend to, so we must not drive them out of the picture to begin with."

But we do attempt to drive them off. When cellular memories become nagging symptoms, the body is attempting to call our attention to something that needs our awareness. Our choice is often to medicate symptoms without meditating on them. Rather than spend time with sensations, we tend to look for ways to avoid them. One problem with this approach is the body's tendency to follow-up on ignored or treated symptoms with even more interesting presentations.

Another, perhaps more important problem, is that we can get so good at overlooking or masking what we may consider to be negative cellular memory that we inadvertently lose sight of even those memories and sensations that feel good.

In order to fully realize the potential value of cellular memory it is important to take this concept two steps further. First, while we appreciate that the body carries memory throughout its "fathomlong" form, we must remember that included within this energetic body library is information regarding the essence of our authenticity. When Jesus said, "The Kingdom of God is within you," I wonder if this is what he was referring to: that everything we need to know, can know, about ourselves already essentially exists in our very cells. As the cellular memories acquired over a human lifetime or lifetimes are acknowledged and released, we begin to uncover other memories of who we truly are.

Secondly, when we begin to remember, when we catch glimpses of our essential nature through sensational moments of love, compassion, beauty or peace, we can begin to add these new memories of such moments to our receptive body tissues. We can develop new banks of memory to be drawn upon during difficult times, which can help us remain present, calm and wise rather than painfully afraid. Intentionally, over time, human emotion and experience become balanced with the sensations and knowledge of spiritual essence.

My experience with long distance backpacking cracked open the doors that I had slammed shut against my body, its sentience and its cellular memory. My experience with Yoga allowed me to slowly and steadily continue to coax these doors open, first revealing what was standing in the way of self-realization and gradually revealing my authentic self.

Yoga, Cellular Memory and Fascia

> *In the practice of Yoga every cell is consciously made to absorb*
> *a copious supply of fresh blood and life-giving energy,*
> *thus satiating the embodied soul.*
>
> — B.K.S. Iyengar

The physical practice of Yoga postures (exercises or asanas) kneads the body's cells, moving energetic information and triggering cellular memories. The silence, invitations to awareness and focused breathing, begin to rouse one's curiosity toward the sensations, thoughts, feelings or images that will inevitably arise. Michael Lee, founder of Phoenix Rising Yoga Therapy, says that in Yoga we are given the opportunity to "meet ourselves through our bodies."

One type of tissue in particular may hold the key to understanding the storage of cellular memory. Fascia is the name given to the vast system of pliable connective tissue that webs its way throughout the body in support of organs, systems and other tissues. It surrounds, spreads within and separates muscles. In some cases, it provides attachments for muscles to bones. Fascia is a connecting medium for almost all of the body.

Massage therapist and Reiki master, Byron Pringer, suggests the concept of "sensory field arrays" – energetic fields consisting of "multiple layers of fascia . . . in varying numbers of planes in any given area of soft tissue." He theorizes that emotions and memories can become stuck in these arrays of fascia, depending on the moisture content/quality of the fascial tissue itself, a process he calls a fascial-based emotional memory storage system.

Pringer's ideas are interesting because it is well known that Yoga asanas *do* manipulate the body's fascial tissue to a great degree. In addition, it is not unusual for memories and feelings to arise when fascia is touched or massaged. All of this might make one wonder if it is in fact fascia that is responsible for holding and releasing held memories and feelings.

In the physical practice of Yoga, intrinsic strength, active flexibility and balance develop as unnatural, fear-based tensions, and samskaras are freed. The developing material body parallels the unveiling of the authentic nature of being. One can come to recognize both humanity and divinity within the process of being embodied. Aspects of human nature become joined or yoked with aspects of divine nature. This union is at the heart of Yoga and, for me, defines authenticity.

I wrote the following poem after two years of consistent Yoga practice and near the end of a week-long intensive Yoga experience. When I read it now, I see it as an example of how my practice eventually deepened my awareness of *both* my human nature and my divine nature:

Sitting With Shame

Shame feels like a hole,
In which fear and sadness sit together
Huddled around the searing flames
Of judgment.

Judgment feeds her own fire,
Rising smoke obliterating
The diamond sky
Of Self-Worth.

Sitting with fear and sadness,
Seek not to push them from the fire's edge,
But rather hold
Their trembling hands.

Be still and wait
Until the flames of judgment
Become the glowing embers
Of compassion.

Invite, then, a clearer upward gaze,
And find
A little bit
Of the shimmering, diamond Self.

Further inquiry into such things as cellular memory and sentience may encounter a few obstacles.

The first obstacle is the locating of something that has no known substance. Memory cannot be touched, seen or captured. It exists, but how? It has the quality of image, yet the actual, tangible image of a memory cannot be viewed by looking at a cell through a microscope. The same can be said of intelligence. We know these things somehow exist. We seem to be able to measure them both, yet what we are measuring we cannot isolate, locate, or fully control.

Another task is one of moving from external to internal, and expansion to integration. The allopathic model of medicine has (admittedly to the benefit of many patients) focused on repairing rather than healing, and specialization rather than holism. As a culture we have demanded external cures to the extent that we have forgotten our intra-personal role of self-healer. Modern medicine has responded, in part, by dividing up the body into areas of specialization, such as podiatry, gynecology and psychiatry.

In order for further study into cellular sentience and memory to occur, it appears that there is a need for an accompanying cultural shift in the direction of whole person care and self-responsibility. In witnessing the upsurge of holistic trends and body-oriented healing modalities in the West today, it appears that this shift is beginning to happen.

In exploring the concepts of cellular intelligence, science will move deeper into the realm of spirituality. I can only imagine the effects such a direction will produce on leading world religious orders and individual belief systems.

Whatever obstacles are met, the possibilities of future science are vast and exciting. In the meantime, what we know now is enough to invite us to continue to explore ourselves within our own bodies – to be our own self-researchers. The inner exploration is always to be continued.

Exercise

This exercise may help you remember how to listen to sensation. A helper will be needed to read the meditation to you. You may find it helpful to speak out loud about your experiences as they unfold during this meditation. This way your helper will know when to continue to the next cue. Stand, close your eyes or soften your gaze toward the floor and allow a few breaths to come and go. When you are ready, invite your helper to begin reading this:

> Turn your attention to a life situation that is presently occupying your attention. *(Pause)* Quite literally, how do you stand in relationship to this situation? *(Pause)* Where in your body, do you feel this relationship – this situation? *(Pause)* What sensations are happening in this place or in these places? What is your actual experience of these sensations? *(Pause)* Over the next few breaths check to see if there is anything else to be explored right now. *(Pause)* Now allow a full breath *(Pause for the breath)* and, as you are ready, keeping your awareness on any sensations you experienced, open your gaze and balance your focus between your sensations from this experience and the next experience of re-entering this room.

Sit for a few minutes and write down what seems important to you about this exercise.

CHAPTER 2

RELATIONSHIP TO THE BODY

What is required (of you) is not perfection but completeness.
— Carl Jung, 1931

I have always been intrigued with my relationship to my body. As I entered more deeply into my practice of body awareness, I watched how I described it in conversation and thought, as well as how I spoke directly to it. I observed how I responded to its sensations. One day I wrote down these leading words in my journal: "My body is . . . ." and quickly completed this sentence in as many ways as I could.

I spoke the words I had written out loud, "My body is . . . . fat, ugly, not good enough, too big, painful, and sinful," and also "strong and basically healthy." I closed *my* eyes and noticed how it felt in my body to say these words. I found that my body felt the way I described it. My words, thoughts and beliefs altered my posture – my presence. As I stayed with my body, some new words came: "My body is sad, hidden, misunderstood" and also "okay the way it is, more than I can easily admit and uniquely wonderful."

It is so easy to consider bodies as objects that are somehow separate from us. Even many of the best Yoga teachers guide students to move or focus on "the legs," "the arms," "the breath," versus using "your" or "my" to describe body parts. And often, when we do use "my" to describe a body part, we do so with the underlying belief that what we are speaking of is actually a separate phenomenon that needs fixing, changing, or some form of objectification or ownership by default, instead of by miracle. We are *we*, and our body is *it*. *It* is something separate from *us*. *We* are either superior to *it* or a slave to *it*.

Certainly, our bodies are related to practicality. They allow us to function in this world of matter. We use, misuse, abuse, disguise, hide, distort, love, hate, judge, flaunt, ignore, avoid, excuse, deny and appreciate our bodies. We are often oblivious to our bodies when they are working well, and we tend to feel angry with, cheated by or disappointed in our bodies, when they appear to be painful burdens that limit our abilities.

I think it is possible to reframe our relationship to body – to reconsider ourselves *as* our bodies and, in doing so, reclaim our responsibilities for self- awareness, self-care and self-healing. As embodied beings what we *must* 'own' is our experience of being embodied.

An Unfortunate Separation

Long ago, flesh and bone became separate from soul and spirit – mind and body were theoretically parted. This separation was enhanced by French biologist and philosopher René Descartes (1596-1650) who put forth the notion that thinking – the refined mind – was separate from the gross body. His 1637 statement "I think, therefore I am" turned thinking into "the real substrate of being" and the body into a purely mechanical process whose sole purpose was to support thinking.

Descartes' research and theory were very much influenced by his relationship with Pope Urban VIII, who had agreed to allow him to study cadavers on the basis that he was only interested in the body apart from the human soul (a task best left to the church). While this agreement between science and religion did open the doors more widely to modern medicine, the body was minimized in the process. Descartes' theory continues to influence Western science and culture today. The word "anatomy" was created — "ana" rooted in "the soul" and "tomy" meaning "to cut from." The science of cutting the soul from the body had begun. As a result, we have become all too casual about the ways in which we split the body from mind, emotion and spirit.

Science said that the body was a marvelous machine to be ruled by the separate mind. In Western culture, religion said that the heart and spirit belonged to God and the church. To varying degrees, we have believed both of them. Even those of us who squirm with discomfort over concepts that keep these aspects of self separate have difficulty finding the language to keep them unified. Helena Norberg Hodge writes, "Indeed, in the West there are so many forces separating spirit, body, and nature that it takes constant effort to live from a deep experiential knowing of interdependence."

A Mechanical Disadvantage

Through the innovations of the Industrial Age and its coinciding medical breakthroughs, we have found it easier and, we thought, more helpful to observe the body's seemingly separate functions as mechanical in nature. Perhaps we have allowed this perspective to remain prevalent because machines are so much easier to understand and explain than bodies. After all, you can take machines apart, find out all there is to know about them, and put them back together. You can fix them when they break and improve them with new parts.

The body-as-machine concept has led us to view the body in at least three distorted ways. The first is our view that the body is a factory comprised of several single-function machines. We assume if one of our inner machines breaks down, we should simply be able to fix just *that one,* and we'll be up and running again. Secondly, because machines were created to do work in the service of man, we've extended these expectations to the body machine, assuming it to be our separate servant. Thirdly, if we consider the body to be mechanical and subservient, then it follows that some part of us must run the machine. Hence the concept of "mind over matter" takes hold while we, at the same time, forget that brain and mind are part of the so-called machine.

I offer a different perspective of body. I suggest that we cannot be considered as simply the sum of our working parts, nor are we somehow independent rulers of our bodies. Consider this: We can easily know who it was who assembled a machine as well as who created each of its parts. We can know what turns it on, what powers it, and how it shuts off. Can we know this about the body?

To Have or to Be?

What happens when we begin to make the shift from having a body to being a body? What if thinking about the body was enhanced by fully experiencing the body? What if we are body? What if we no longer needed to search outside of ourselves for something to make us happy? What if happiness is already inside right now?

And, if the body is "the sage within the temple" and not merely the temple, are we willing to be the sages that we are? Are there, perhaps, responsibilities to self and others that we would need to acknowledge if we were to recognize ourselves as sages? How might that change us? How might it change the world?

Weeks after doing the exercise of writing the words "My body is . . ." in my journal, I tried a different approach. I wrote the words, "I am . . ." in place of "My body is . . ." from the previous exploration. It felt both odd and right to recognize that in describing my body I was describing myself, both personally and in a somewhat broader context. "I" was not separate from "body" unless some aspect of me chose to create the illusion that "I" was so.

I also discovered that the descriptive words I wrote and spoke had a much greater impact when they were related to "I." In this way, I could not dump my perceived limitations on a seemingly other thing – my body – in much the same way I might disparage another person behind their back. I was saddened by the realization of how I disparaged myself. I was also more determined to increase my awareness of this in all areas of my life, to look deeply at why this so easily happened and to wonder about being in a different, more compassionate relationship with myself.

Forgetting and Remembering

My body
You are so kind to sit
And wait for me
While I'm away

I wander off
But you don't budge
When I return to my true home
It is you

— Casey Hayden

Somewhere along the road of life we begin to forget what we knew as infants. We are embodied consciousness – both human and divine. Babies and small children seem to know this. They live through discovering the physical miracle that they are, and they naturally assume their own perfection. They express their emotions fully at the appropriate time. Babies marvel in their uniqueness and understand connectedness. They do not consider their mistakes to be failures. If a baby were to react to mistakes with the same amount of self-judgment that we have as adults, he or she would most likely never learn to walk.

Our separateness is an essential aspect of development in human society. It is encouraged according to our cultural family, and, in comparison to that family, we see our imperfections and differences. We begin to judge ourselves and set ourselves up to play our roles in life the best way we can. As we awaken to our assumptions of what life and culture seem to expect of us, we fall asleep when it comes to body and the reality of who we are. In that sleep, however, we dream. We have a distant clouded memory of what we knew as infants. We begin to notice the possible discrepancy between our *concepts* of who we think we are and the actual *felt awareness* of ourselves.

When something happens in your body, when some new or unusual sensation occurs, it would make sense to be curious about it. It would seem as though you might want to pay attention to it and learn more about its reasons for being there. However, most of us do not move into sensation with genuine curiosity and attention. Instead, we try to turn down or turn off the sensational music of the body, and, to a certain degree, the body complies. Eventually, however, having our best interest at heart, body will find creative ways to turn its volume back up, often demanding attention in ways we no longer can ignore. When this happens, we have the opportunity to discover that it is harder to bear the costs of avoiding the body than it is to experience any discomfort that might accompany its deeper exploration. As Emerson wrote, "When a dog is chasing after you, whistle for him.."

At some point, distracted by the "dog" and drawn by the instinct that there is something to us that is somehow missing, many of us sincerely turn in the direction of distant memory, moving slowly toward it as if it were a candle burning in the corner of a dark room. I suggest that we can turn toward our bodies as one way back to that light.

Clearly, the process I describe above is not a negative one. It is part and parcel of the human experience to spiral through knowing, forgetting and remembering. One phenomenon supports the other. Who knows? Perhaps forgetting is a process that is crucial in order for consciousness to become conscious of itself. What we tend to also forget is that all of this happens in the body – by way of the body – whether we are aware of it or not. Separation and forgetting happen in the body. Enlightenment and awakening happen in the body. The body is the happening place!

Becoming Bilingual – Learning Sensational Language

The mindful individual learns to listen to every cell in his bodymind and to be responsive to its needs and lessons.
— Ken Dychtwald

My mentor and friend, Karen Hasskarl, often says, "There is no such thing as a purely physical experience." By this she means that every physical experience is also somehow emotional, intellectual and spiritual. Along the same lines we could say that there is no such thing as a purely emotional experience, or a purely intellectual one, and maybe not even a purely spiritual one.

When I think a thought, I cannot accurately pinpoint in my body where that thought came from. I assume that it comes from my head, although I have been taught that my brain is in my skull, and thought comes from my brain, alone. The more I draw my awareness toward the source of thought, the more thought feels like a whole-body experience interwoven with emotion and sensation.

Exercise

Begin by playing some music that is moving, energetic or otherwise inspirational. Stand still and notice where in your body any movement wants to begin. Notice any longing to move or resistance to moving. After a few moments, allow your body to begin to move the way it wants to. At first, keep the movements small, local and as subtle as a flower's bud opening it petals. Allow the movement to emerge from the inside out. Gradually let your movement intensify, *your* rhythm playing with the rhythm of the music. Notice the parts of your body that are fully participating, as well as the parts that are more reluctant. After dancing for a few minutes, notice any emotions that are arising, and any thoughts that accompany your movement. As the music ends, turn off the machine that has been playing it, and stand very still. In this space of silence, turn your focus toward any experiences that are occurring inside you right now, as well as any that seem to be somehow absent. Notice the energy of *being* in your body. Catch a glimpse of the sensation of *being* – of your essence. To whatever extent is possible right now, contact the humming essence of life inside your body.

To me, it feels like coming home to my whole self. I can no longer say that dance is a purely physical experience separate from feeling, thought and self-essence.

The language of sensation is one that we all know, yet we forget how to speak it. We forget that sensation accompanies all aspects of self, as we move through life. Life circumstances come and go, and we rarely stop and consult with the sensational aspects of thought and emotion, which by far offer the most honest and accurate information on which to base life decisions.

Interpreting the Language of the Body: Stepping into the Metaphysical Without Tripping

The body begins to form itself around the feelings that animate it,
and the feelings, in turn, become habituated
and trapped within the body tissue itself.
— Ken Dychtwald

The term "metaphysical" is loosely linked to the word "metaphorical." If something is metaphysical, it is considered to be somehow related to a philosophy of ultimate reality, which is thought to somehow be beyond matter or physical nature. One can apply concepts that seem to be psychological or philosophical to things which are assumed to be physical. In this way a metaphysical concept is somewhat like a metaphorical one in which a term or trait that is normally assigned to one thing is attached to another thing as a way of comparison, explanation or correspondence.

Bodies, sensations and posture are often interpreted through theories of tissue correspondences, character armor and the *seven chakras*. The concept of tissue correspondences refers to the types of energy that have become associated with various types of body tissue and to body areas. Postural discrepancies which, according to Western psychology, tend to accompany certain aspects of personality are commonly referred to as character armor. And the seven chakras are the vertically oriented centers in the human body that correspond to human needs and evolutionary process.

I mention tissue types and chakras because they are prevalent in our culture's current stream of information regarding the search for self. Visit any bookstore's "New Age" section, and you will find an abundant amount of material on these subjects. I include the character perspective because it has eventually led the West in the direction of understanding cellular memory and dharma. While each perspective has value, reliance on one or a combination of these concepts is to adopt assumptions about one's own experience of body. Such assumptions can stand in the way of actual sensation and its individual truth.

Metaphysical perspectives can be useful for making interesting comparisons and for spurring self-questioning. They also may provide a starting point for the continued observation of sensation, but they should not be considered absolute prescriptions for predicting the root of sensation or type of experience.

However, there is a value to briefly touching on each concept as a way of deepening the understanding of the potential dharma of sentient tissues and the vast possibilities of cellular memory.

Tissue Types and Correspondences

The concept of tissue types is, in part, based on the "principle of correspondences" suggested by Robert St. John and Emanuel Swendenborg, which states that "Every natural physical manifestation has a relationship to corresponding non-physical states of being or principle." In other words, every body experience/sensation corresponds to an already established, universally experienced collective meaning represented by the area of the body that is the center for that experience/sensation. Much in the same way that dream images can be related to archetypal symbols of the collective unconscious, areas of the body are associated with certain universal meanings.

For example, according to the system of thought surrounding tissue correspondences, our backs are the places we store all of the aspects of ourselves that we don't want to see, such as guilt. Pain in the back may also be related to a need for some sort of support. Even more specifically, pain in the upper back is thought to be related to emotional support, while low back discomfort is believed to connect to financial support. Some other examples of tissue types and their corresponding metaphysical elements are: bone represents spiritual energy, blood and other body fluids correspond to emotional energy, feet have to do with foundation, knees have to do with progress, muscle is representative of mental energy and colons are representative of holding on to the past.

In general, such correspondences often have a ring of truth, and as we explore our bodies for sensory information, we may well discover what we experience somehow fits into the picture suggested by universal tissue types. Joints, for instance, are about connection. I could most definitely agree that my Long Trail shoulder pain corresponded to my disconnection to the burden (shoulder related) of grief that I was carrying.

Here's the catch: If we depend on the theory of correspondences as the all-case truth, or if we predict the outcome of our awareness by relying on their assumptions, we are coming to sensation with expectations generated by others and an outside-in approach to self-discovery. This may ultimately get in the way of noticing the reality of in-the-moment sensation and its often unique meanings.

Months after my hike, while sitting in meditation, I gained a much deeper awareness of my then chronic shoulder discomfort. I received an image of my body as a rag doll. In this image, my affected arm had been sewn in too tightly. My actual sensation was that I was drawn in at that shoulder joint. The corresponding personal metaphor was protection rather than connection. While my previous correspondences with connection and burden were far from incorrect, my deeper realization about protection was more to the point and more uniquely meaningful.

Character Armor and the Psychology of Muscle

Character armor concepts are rooted in Western psychology's early assumptions of character analysis. From Charles Darwin to Wilhelm Reich and from Sigmund Freud to Alexander Lowen, assumptions about posture and neurosis were constructed. Their case was this: "On the psychic level [whatever and wherever that is] certain thoughts (are prevented) from reaching consciousness, so on a biological level (whatever this is), spastic, chronically contracted muscles prevent certain impulses from reaching the surface." Lowen and his predecessors postulated that specific posture traits would likely correspond to various abnormal character types such as oral, masochistic, hysterical, phallic-narcissistic, passive-feminine, schizophrenic and schizoid types. According to this approach to body, an oral character, having been deprived of nurturing as an infant, would appear immature with poorly developed muscles, a generally weak sunken posture, thin skin, flat feet, a forward tilted head, collapsed chest and a softly protruding abdomen. Whew!

To some extent it is true that posture *is* created according to our beliefs and expectations about ourselves and our environments. Posture does tend to reflect our coping strategies for living in the world. However, while these early concepts of embodied experience were useful to the diagnosis and treatment of mental illness and perhaps marked the beginning of a return to valuing the body as an essential element of transformation, if you come in contact with this approach to your own body, I suggest that you follow this advice: "Run!" Run fast and far away from these assumptions, which will have you permanently sleeping on your analyst's couch, worrying about what is wrong with you. Attachment to the negative stereotypes of character analysis severely limits the truth of direct experience, especially for those of us who are not clinically mentally ill.

An outgrowth of character analysis which is parallel to Eastern thinking and quite helpful to the process of self-understanding is called by psychologist James Gavin "the psychology of muscle." Gavin and others, such as Ken Dykwald and Ron Kurtz, softened the extreme views of abnormal character traits, taking from this early approach ideas that were more applicable to understanding normally functioning human bodies. What Gavin says can be considered another, perhaps broader, version of tissue correspondences, which seems to relate fairly well to the experience of many Yoga movements and exercises.

Consider your arms and hands . . . how they push things away and pull things in. They gather, touch, caress, hit, make or avoid contact and help you with balance. They are the part of you that enables you to *do* practical things. This is an example of the psychology of muscle. Notice, however, that we are talking about whole arms – muscle, bone, joint, connective tissue, blood, nerves etc.

I have found that, especially during Yoga practice, the metaphors surrounding my arms, legs and other body parts help me to experience myself in interesting ways. The following exercise is a simple example.

Exercise

Stand facing a wall and place your hands on it at shoulder height and width, then step backward until you can straighten your elbows. Take one more step back with both feet so your whole body is now slightly angled toward the wall, elbows still straight, let your weight move in toward the wall through your straightened arms. Begin to notice if your sensation is of trying to push the wall. Or is the wall pushing *you* . . . or perhaps supporting you? What is it like to push . . to be pushed . . . to be supported? What other parts of your body are speaking-up in relation to this experience? What is happening with your breath? The longer you remain in this position, what things are changing? How are they changing? What thoughts, emotions or images arise? Are there any current or historical life circumstances from which you experience or remember similar sensations? Or are there any in which you would like to experience these sensations?

You can learn a great deal through your body about yourself by doing simple movements such as this, and becoming curious about all you notice in the process.

The Seven Chakras

According to Yoga philosophy, particularly that of Tantric, Kundalini and Hatha Yoga, the seven chakra centers of the human body represent the "axis mundi" or "the central axis of the world that runs through the vertical core of each one of us." Each chakra (literally translated as "wheel" or "disc") is considered to be a center of activity of life force energy. At each of the seven areas from our tailbones to the crowns of our heads is said to exist a "spinning sphere of bioenergetic activity" or "wheel of becoming" that is related to the nerve bundles that extend from our spinal chords out into these regions.

According to Yoga traditions, Shakti, the manifested female aspect of divinity, is thought to reside near the base of our vertical chakra line. Shiva, her male, yet to be manifested counterpart, is thought to dwell in waiting for Shakti at the crown top of the chakra line. The serpent power of Kundalini energy rises in a spiral manner up our spines as Shakti energy tries to unite with Shiva energy. The evolution and condition of our chakra centers either allow or interrupt this flow of divine energy.

The chart on the next page represents, in a very general way, the basic aspects of the chakra system. Again, I have both respect and appreciation for the wisdom behind this ancient philosophy as well as hesitations concerning their overuse as a transformative guide. I find discussions on the chakra centers fascinating and full of potential for deeper self-questioning and understanding. I also think that too much reliance on the observation of these centers can limit individual discovery of truth in the same way that categorizing character according to posture/armor analysis limits one's ability to discover one's own reality.

Reliance on such systems or categories can lead one to *expect* to find certain conditions, weaknesses or strengths and assumes a level of judgment as to whether or not these aspects of self are bad or good. There is a sense of "should" behind the teachings of the chakra centers, although when employed as a general guide, the information that is offered through its teachings can form a valuable base from which to deepen self-awareness.

The concepts of cellular sentience, cellular memory and correspondences intertwine and overlap in much the same way that the miraculous body network does. It is helpful to return to the multi-dimensional perspective of the whole body and remember that no one cell or system is independent of the others. Perhaps entwining the principals of correspondences, chakras and personal continued awareness is the best broad approach to self-discovery. However, it is also helpful to remember that first and foremost, the most reliable and truthful information that can be gathered about oneself exists in one's own body.

While outer authorities are helpful and worth consideration, we must ultimately look inside for the present truth. As Patañjali's Yoga sutra 1.7 suggests, "Understanding arises from sensory perception, inference, and faithful testimony . . . right knowledge is obtained through direct observation."

A BASIC REPRESENTATION OF THE SEVEN CHAKRA CENTERS

Energetic Center	Correspondence To Body	Qualities	Urges & Intentions	Energetic Goals/Risks
Shiva Energy	Above The Head	Male, Unmanifested, Spirit	Transcending Body	Union with Shakti
7th Chakra	Crown of The Head	Awareness, Wisdom, Unity-Consciousness	Love of Self (or God)	To Know, Spiritual Connection
6th Chakra	Forehead, Between the eyebrows	Intuition, Psychic perception, Understanding	Love Of Life	To See Clearly, Self-Reflection
5th Chakra	Throat	Communication, Expression, Resonance	Love Of Truth	To Speak, To be Heard
4th Chakra	Heart	Self-acceptance, Love, Compassion, Relationship, Balance	Love of Being in The World	To Love, To be Loved
3rd Chakra	Solar Plexus to Belly Button	Self-esteem, Power, Will, Purpose, Vitality	The Will To Be/Act	To Act, To Seek Identity
2nd Chakra	Abdomen, Genitals, Lower Back, Hips	Sexuality, Pleasure, Passion, Self-Gratification	The Will To Feel	To Want, To Feel
1st Chakra	Base of Spine	Survival, Self-Preservation, Trust	The Will To Live	To be Here, To Have
Shakti	At and Beneath The Base of the Spine	Female, Manifested, Earth	Grounded	Union With Shiva

CHAPTER 3
ATTEMPTING TO DEMYSTIFY CONSCIOUSNESS

There are things in the psyche which I do not produce,
but which produce themselves and have their own life.

— Carl Jung

The words "consciousness" and "conscious" and their presumptive partners "unconsciousness" and "unconscious" have frequently mystified me. The concepts these terms represent are difficult to understand and awkward to assimilate into daily experience. I have yet to discover any Western or Eastern text that provides me with absolute clarity concerning the concept of consciousness. Even though we have been asking questions of this phenomenon for thousands of years, we still find ourselves supposing what it is. I'm not at all sure that clarity is possible.

I don't have to know if I am right or wrong about consciousness. For me to unfold my personal journey feels more important than knowing. However, some level of discussion about consciousness seems essential to my proposal that the body is deeply involved in the process of self-revelation and transformation. Though it may or may not be possible to fully understand consciousness, I do believe body awareness might provide us with our best chance to do so. It is through the body that we experience, to varying degrees, the presence of consciousness.

Consciousness as Energetic Unifier

Where does the body end and the mind begin?
Where does the mind end and the spirit begin?
They cannot be divided as they are interrelated and but different
aspects of the same all-pervading divine consciousness.

— B.K.S. Iyengar

From my journal, May 2002:

Practice today . . . gentle Yoga asanas and a walking meditation. I notice how in walking meditation there is a sense of watching myself and a sense of moving too slowly. This is not always the case (the moving too slowly part that is). I do watch myself. I realize when I am alone, I view my movements, actions, thoughts, as if I were outside of me. I have trouble pulling myself inside. Who is the one who is watching? Am I the watcher? Or am I the watched. Or am I the one who watches the watcher and the watched? Or am I all of these?

The one who is doing is hesitant. She is the adolescent who cares too much about what her peers think of her. But something in her just wants to be left alone to 'be'. Something in her wants the watcher to 'Fuck off', and yet she is easily overpowered by another part that says, 'Aren't you looking at me? Don't you notice me? Am I not someone? Aren't I beautiful? Don't I do this well? Please tell me I am worthy of your attention.'

The watcher says, 'Nobody's looking at you. You are invisible. You mean nothing. Look how you try to stand out. You should be ashamed. Who do you think you are, desiring to be watched? Everyone will be thinking the worst if they see you.'

The "one who watches the watcher *and* the watched" does not interfere. She loves them both. She understands them both. She waits for a future balance of power and humility, of grace and light, of receiving and giving, of having and not needing, of open awareness and honest appraisal. But she knows that these two – the watcher and the watched need to exist. This One – the observer – waits.

Carl Jung, father of Jungian psychotherapy, student of Yoga and fellow searcher for the human soul, describes consciousness as a "common psychic [energetic] substrate of a suprapersonal nature, which is present in every one of us." Psychologist and explorer of the Yoga sutras (rules for being) Geraldine Coster suggested that consciousness is "the perceiver, the act of perceiving and the thing being perceived" all at the same time. Developmental psychologist Robert Kegan refers to it as "a kind of species sympathy, which we do not share so much as it shares us."

From the perspective of Yoga, consciousness or, more accurately, "Being-Consciousness" is the supreme Absolute, the unique Knowledge, the everlasting Tranquility – the unique "space of Awareness." It is essential, formative energy. As fascia interconnects all aspect of a body, the web of consciousness interconnects all things.

One enjoys liberation when one knows that the Self is the Witness,
the Truth, the Whole, all pervasive, nondual, supreme,
and though abiding in the body is not body bound.
— From the *Mahnirvana Tantra* 14.116.135

Yoga psychology suggests that consciousness is the aware energy that creates our universe and all things in it. Its impulse is to become matter, which indicates that it is something apart from matter as well. It is energy in material form as well as energy that is somehow yet to be manifested. Once it inhabits matter, its impulse is to know itself again as immaterial pure consciousness. It is both the tangible, less subtle matter of a thing as well as the less tangible, very subtle essence of that same thing.

Consciousness as a Level of Awareness

Consciousness as a level of awareness describes the quality and quantity of normal waking state. It is the term used to speak about one's usual, day-to-day "pattern of cognitive, perceptual, emotional [embodied] functioning." At any given moment we are more or less aware (conscious) of ourselves within our surroundings. To varying degrees, we perceive and understand our current experience. we also perceive what *might* be happening based on my prior experiences with similar situations. And our awareness carries forward into the possibilities of the future as well as to any number of other things that may or may not be directly related to the situation at hand. Our attention is sometimes narrow and focused and other times broad and expanding.

We experience awareness as embodied thought, sensation and emotion. For instance, right now I am writing. I know I am writing because I feel my fingers on the keyboard and my eyes are seeing the words appear on my computer screen. I am reading and, at the same time, thinking about the best way to write what I want to say. I feel the energy of my passion for this subject in my heart and belly. I notice that my upper back is tense from sitting at the computer. I am aware of the underlying body-wide sensations of the stress of having a deadline. I notice that I am beginning to feel hungry and that my feet are cold. I remember I need to call my sister and we need eggs for breakfast tomorrow. All of this and more falls into my present frame of awareness as I keep on typing.

It can be astonishing to sit down and make a list of everything that you are aware of at any one moment. If you ask, "What else?" there is usually something more to add to the list. Each moment brings new awareness even when you don't think there is much going on. As the moments pass and awareness shifts, it is interesting to notice the thoughts, sensations and emotions that are either somehow present or perhaps strangely absent.

By exploring moment by moment awareness in this way, I began to see the width and breadth of my potential to be conscious (aware). As I learned how to explore my body for information about myself, I was equally surprised to discover the extent to which I had previously been unaware. I began to wonder; could it be that I was somehow imposing my own limits on my ability to be conscious? If so, why would I do this? Looking deeper, I discovered how old habits and self-beliefs kept this sort of consciousness from expanding in certain directions. I was able to control and direct my awareness.

Awareness of Energy

As we progress and awaken to the soul in us and things,
we shall realize that there is a consciousness also in the plant,
in the metal, in the atom, in electricity,
in everything that belongs to physical nature.

— Sri Aurobindo

I am drawn to "everyday miracles" – those not so unusual events that ground us with a felt sensation of unified energy or understanding. For example, just yesterday I brought some flowering plants back into the house from the front porch. It's October and the frosts have begun. I placed one plant in a sunny window, its purple blossoms facing into the room so I could enjoy them only to find that a short time later all those blossoms had turned outward to face the sun again. In that brief moment when I realized that this non-human thing had some human-like intention, had consciously turned toward its source of life, I felt a kind of awe, bliss and recognition. For a moment I felt as if I were somehow a part of that plant's beauty. I instantly understood why it had turned. No explanation was necessary. I knew because I would have done the same thing, for the same reason. The plant and I shared some cross-species knowledge, some level of awareness.

Everyday miracles such as this occur all the time. We need only be awake enough to catch them as they happen. It is easier to take notice of the bigger ones. Those of us who have participated in the birth of a child will remember the joyous sensations of *that* moment. Those who have witnessed the death of any living thing will never forget the sensations received through another's passing. These experiences are *bigger,* but not so far *different* from the eagerness of a plant turning toward the sun, or the time-stopping landing of a dragonfly on my knee or the sound of crunching snow under my winter, full-moon footstep.

The sensations of joy, love and unity connected to everyday miracles are felt in the body. These are the sensations of embodying the energy of consciousness.

One dramatic but certainly everyday miracle is found in watching the progress of a beautiful sunset until its end. I have done this many times from mountain tops as well as my own front porch. Facing west and watching the inevitable ending of the day, I sometimes get the sense that I am participating – that it is possible for me to *see* the beauty of this sunset because I *am* that same beauty. For a few seconds I see the reflection of my essence in the colors across the sky. A witness of the sunset, I allow the possibility that "observer and observed are not ultimately distinct."

To acknowledge such a possibility feels both impossible and real. I feel the beauty of the sunset in the center of my chest. It is not an emotion. It is a feeling of knowing beauty – of being it. It is a feeling of identification and relationship. I sense where *I* am, and I understand where the *sun* is setting, but is there really a separation between the two of us? For a few moments my answer is, "No." Later on, I tend to forget. However, memory of this miracle has landed in my cells. When the next one occurs, I might experience the event more *in* me than *around* me.

Everyday miracles provide us with chances to become *conscious* of the unitary nature of *consciousness*, itself. How would we be able to do this without our body? Just as personal experiences happen in each body, so does the experience of being consciousness. The sensations of unity I experience seem set in harmony with and balanced by, the parallel reality of my individual, unique human nature. I seem to need to be separate in order to experience connection.

Feuerstein writes, "Existence is an infinitely complex network of conditions giving rise to other conditions." This quote reads just as eloquently if I change "Existence" to "My body." Through witnessing my body in relationship to events I get to experience something more of the "vast . . . organizing field of existence." I step in the direction of self — the inherent, grounding presence of consciousness and the uniquely beautiful details of my personal story.

Before my Long Trail Adventure, I had become accustomed to viewing consciousness primarily as the extent to which I was aware of myself separate from the world. I had lost contact with the broader context of consciousness and, therefore, of myself. By losing contact with self, self called to be remembered. And, almost as soon as I asked the question, "Who am I really?," I began to experience what my mentor Karen Hasskarl calls "the deep unknowing of the familiar" — a relearning of the delicate balance (union) of individuality and unity.

By being bodies rather than possessing bodies, by recognizing body as a valuable source of knowledge, we are able, once again, to become familiar with the subtly felt essence of the vastness of consciousness. At the same time, we can experience the felt sensations of being matter. The body links the memory of the one consciousness (totality) to the rich diversity of being human. We are "differentiated unity." To cut oneself off from one's body is to sever the knowledge of both these aspects of consciousness (individual and unitary), which together form the true self.

This differentiated unity is felt and, for me, understood in the arc of tension between energy and matter. I notice this arc between the soles of my feet and the top of my head, between my right and left sides, between my front and back surfaces, between the intrinsic opposing spirals of my spinal column, between me and other individuals, and between me and surrounding nature. It seems that these tension arcs hold energy and matter together as one unitary thing.

A Collective Perspective

> *The world is our true body.*
> — Georg Feuerstein

> *I am the truth from foot to brow.*
> — Rumi

Consciousness is both personal and transpersonal. It is held both individually and in common (universally/collectively). It has an integrative tendency and seeks harmony and completion. Because we are beings of this same energy, we, too, seek these same things and long to integrate our separate uniqueness into the world community, to yoke or union with other focal points of consciousness and ultimately, if only for a moment now and then, with the felt energy of consciousness itself.

Consciousness is naturally unitary, eternal, unencumbered, impartial, ever-present, wise, loving and compassionate. These same qualities are at the heart of human authenticity. To a large degree, they describe the natural self I have been in search of. Recognizing the nature of consciousness as an important aspect of my *own* true nature, while still appreciating those qualities that make me unique, is a goal of Yoga.

The God Factor (Inevitable Territory)

> *The paradox is that the more deeply we penetrate*
> *the phenomenal world (the body, the earth) with our attention,*
> *the more we discover that the world and its forms*
> *are full of God – indeed, are God,*
> *or more accurately from the Yogic point of view,*
> *God and Goddess.*
>
> — Stephen Cope

Because consciousness has qualities and intentions it is easy to imagine it is an entity that is separate from and more powerful than humans and other beings of matter. Traditionally, cultures attribute human characteristics to what or whom this so-called entity is imagined to be. Hence, God is created by man.

I do not pretend to *know* if consciousness *is* God or Goddess in the traditional sense, nor do I carry any judgment or intend any insult to those who believe in a separate from human – probably male – God, but when I hear that word, "God," I hear the word "*consciousness*" in its place. God and Goddess within my frame of awareness are masculine and feminine qualities of the one energy of consciousness.

I understand and personally feel occasional longings for consciousness to be God/Goddess because I, too, sometimes desire to be comforted, soothed and cared for by such an entity. But then I remember I am made of and held in the wide web of all encompassing consciousness, bound into the fascia of the universe. From my belief that I am a unique and integral representation of consciousness, an even greater comfort arises. If consciousness is divine, then so am I and everything else. Yet, from this perspective, my human individuality, however impermanent it is, is not lost in a sea of transpersonal, transcendent energy, but rather validated as a necessary contribution to the entire community of life and energy.

"All life experiences are the play of the same One," says Feuerstein. While there may be no *energetic* difference between all-encompassing consciousness and that which is integrated into the material world as me, I sense an individual responsibility in being a focal point or hot spot of this one energy. I see the importance of becoming increasingly aware of the ways in which I disrupt the flow of divine energy. If I do so in myself, I affect all other areas of the web. I can discover such disruptions through my body. I can increase my awareness of consciousness by observing and learning from my ebb and flow of sensation, thought and emotion.

If we are focal points of one consciousness, this may explain why we seem to share memory and empathy across cultures and time. Maybe the fascia of consciousness links past and present moments to future ones. As threads of the web, we may all be living the same old story in a never before told, well-known, new way. As psychologist Clyde Ford suggests, "It's as though we are all reading the same conscious book, unconsciously." The body is the great book that we get to read. "For the ignorant person, this body is a source of endless suffering, but to the wise person, this body is a source of infinite delight" (from *Yoga-Vsishtha* 4.23.18.24).

Born Divine – Me? No. You're Just Saying That.

Within the city of Brahman, which is the body, there is the heart,
and within the heart there is a little house.
This house has the shape of a lotus,
and within it dwells that which is to be sought after,
inquired about, and realized.
Even so large as the universe outside is
the universe within the lotus of the heart.
Within it are heaven and earth, the sun, moon,
the lightning and all the stars.
Whatever is in the macrocosm is in this microcosm also.
— From the *Chandogya Upanishad,*
one of the oldest of some 108 Hindu sacred texts of
revelations and metaphysics (dated approximately 2000 BCE)

Consciousness is divine in that its qualities are similar to those attributed to Gods or Goddesses, such as creative power, absolute love, wisdom and compassion. If we are focal points of consciousness, we too have such qualities at the heart of our being. We are "born divine" and, according to our role in the web of all things, can understand that in regards to our life in this world "everything is already okay."

These concepts invited me to take two leaps of faith. One is that I have come to view all that has happened to me and my current situation as valuable, purposeful and "okay." The other is that I am willing to be divine.

It is not an easy thing to consider the pain and struggle of life as okay. Of course, I want to avoid suffering and its costs. This is especially true when I am particularly close to the pains and discomforts of circumstances and events. Yet I have to confess I have found teachers within the trials of life after some time has passed. The greater my understanding of consciousness, which tells me everything is the way it should be, the greater my ability to self-mentor and self-sooth my way through the difficult times of my humanness.

This said, I think it is also important not to remain stuck in suffering mode because it is the right place to be! In accepting that all experience has value, I also accept the implied responsibility to learn and move on.

The second leap of faith involves removing barriers to the concept that I am already divinely complete. As I work to integrate the loose ends of my human experience toward meaning, I attempt to remember that I already possess the seeds of the qualities of consciousness, even if they are not yet cultivated. Even though I now grasp the truth of this, there are times when my Baptist upbringing says I should feel guilty for imagining such a thing. To think that I possess the qualities of God must be blasphemy. I was brought up to de-activate any positive information regarding myself. I did not learn how to receive. I longed for others to substantiate my worthiness, but I found it difficult to take in positive feedback without discounting it. I heard "You look especially beautiful today!" and immediately said to myself "No, I don't. You're just being nice." I heard "You are divine and complete as you are right now!" and my initial response was "Others may be divine, but how could I possibly be?"

My unwillingness to recognize myself as divine was linked to the depths of my personal history, which I had, to varying degrees, suppressed or repressed. This information stood in the way of my ability to know my individual sacredness.

From my journal, February 7, 2002 (following a Yoga class):

> *I notice how hard it is for me to accept attention from others, and yet I crave it. Why? I need/want love, support, recognition . . . but I'm not sure where to put it, when I get it. It's like trying to put the laundry away, when all the drawers are already full. What are my drawers full of? Full of business – so I don't have time to look at what's hidden near the bottom of my drawers? I think it might be shame in there, but I'm not sure. Whatever it is, it has to do with secrets and something to do with not being worthy. My heart knows I am worthy, and other parts of me aren't sure – need time. The courage it takes to look in the drawer is different from the courage needed to clean it out.*

Four days south of the Canadian border when I was end-to-ending the Long Trail, I settled in for a cozy night at Whiteface Mountain shelter. I pitched my tent, took care of housekeeping particulars and kicked back to read the entries in the shelter log, a sort of hiker's guest book of those who had stayed there before me. I opened it to the most recent entry:

> *Our deepest fear is not that we are inadequate. Our deepest fear is that we are powerful beyond measure. It is our light, not our darkness, that frightens us. We ask ourselves, "Who am I to be brilliant, gorgeous, talented and fabulous?" Actually, who are you not to be?*

Note: Although Nelson Mandela used these words in his 1994 Inaugural Address, they are originally attributed to Marianne Williamson.

Yoga philosopher, Joseph Vrinte, writes about this fear of our own greatness – of making ourselves less sacred than we are – as a "desacralizing mechanism." We mistrust the possibility of our divinity or are unwilling to see ourselves as sacred and therefore often refuse to treat ourselves with due respect. But as philosopher Erasmus said, "Invoked or not invoked, the God will be present." Whether or not we acknowledge ourselves as divine, we are.

Coincidently, it was not long after reading the Williamson quote in the trail log that I began to experience the deep pain of holding back grief, which I mentioned earlier. I have often wondered what part the reading of this quote played in the enhancement of my long slow process of self-awareness. While re-reading my Long Trail journal, the second part of the same quote moved into the foreground of my awareness:

> *You are a child of God [You are a focal point of the One Consciousness]. Your playing small doesn't serve the world. There's nothing enlightened about shrinking so that other people won't feel insecure around you. We were born to manifest the glory of God [the totality of consciousness] that is within us. It's not*

just in some of us; it's in everyone. And as we let our light shine, we unconsciously [or consciously] give other people permission to do the same. As we are liberated from our fear, our presence automatically liberates others.

Enter: The Unconscious

The bearer of evil tidings,
When he was halfway there,
Remembered that evil tidings
Were a dangerous thing to bear.

So when he came to the parting
Where one road led to the throne
And one went off to the mountains
And into the wild unknown,
He took the one to the mountains.

— Robert Frost
from his poem, *The Bearer of Evil Tidings*

The concepts of the unconscious or of unconsciousness are also complex. These terms refer to the day-to-day *lack of* awareness and understanding about self and the world. They represent those existent things of which I am, at the moment, unaware. Therefore, the unconscious is associated with the dark underworld of the unknown. On the other hand, it may also be considered as the river of instinctive energy and collective memory of consciousness that connects us to each other through dreams, fairy tales and personal stories.

In defining these aspects of awareness lies the assumption that *un*consciousness is a different thing from consciousness. But one might consider the unconscious as a way of relating to consciousness. The degree to which I am conscious or unconscious of certain things is a measure of my in-the-moment ability to recognize myself as a unique expression of consciousness.

I come into each Yoga practice with my metaphorical backpack full of a certain amount of the stuff of life. Depending on my human situation at the time, I am more or less aware of the quality of energy in my body. At the earlier stages of my practice, I sometimes have a more difficult time remembering the broader view of who I am. I find it much easier to identify primarily with the contents of the pack rather than with the wisdom of consciousness. As I progress through postures, questioning and observing sensation, aspects of my body call me to draw certain items out of the pack for deeper examination. Some things become discarded (appreciated but no longer needed), while others hang around the Yoga mat for a while longer. Some things go back in the pack. And still there are things inside that I am not yet ready to pull out (unconscious things).

As this process continues, I begin to feel the empty spaces in my backpack – in my body. As my relationship to my personal stories shifts and changes, my awareness of the consciousness that inhabits those empty spaces grows. What *is* changing is my ability to integrate the empty space with the stuff of life, to remember my divine nature and validate my human one.

An Unfortunate Reputation

> *Perhaps all the dragons of our lives are princesses*
> *who are only wanting to see us once beautiful and brave.*
> *Perhaps everything terrible is in its deepest being*
> *something helpless that wants help from us.*
> — Rainer Maria Rilke

The unconscious is frequently conceptualized as that place we go down into to discover things that we are not so sure we want to discover. The unconscious becomes as if it were a place, and this place feels very real when we are working toward understanding the depths of our own souls. In fact, it is real. The depths of our unconscious exist in the tissues of our bodies. As embodied beings we are invited to explore the down and dirty things of our human experience, as well as the light and flowing remembrances of consciousness.

The unconscious (the body) is commonly believed to contain information that is too uncomfortable or too difficult to bring into full acknowledged awareness. It is the material of life experience that is somehow "not compatible with the consciousness [way of being in the world] that is being constructed [by an individual at the present time]." Material that is outside of our present moment zone of comfort waits in the unconscious, so that we might be able to cope within the context of our world. This is not a bad thing. This self-protective nature of the unconscious (the body) supports us to survive many current in-the-world situations.

Perhaps it is partly due to this protective nature that the unconscious (and also the body) has gained the reputation for being unknown, hidden and foreboding. We too often view it with negativity or suspicion, assuming that whatever is buried there will be too harmful or rather too *truthful* for us to bear.

If the information we choose to store in ourselves is harmful to us, why would we choose to store it? Perhaps we store information because we know that it has value, that it will somehow one day lead us to self-revelation. Like the family heirloom that I will one day fix up and display on my wall, the material of the unconscious gathers dust and waits.

My sense is that we have no intention of springing horrible information on ourselves. The material we choose, at one time for appropriate reasons, to store in our bodies has the potential to enlighten us, its related discomforts not too overwhelming. We are not apt to push ourselves toward revelation until we are somewhat ready to go there. Buddhist Pema Chödrön writes in her recent book, *The Places That Scare You,* "A first step is to understand that a feeling of dread or psychological discomfort might just be a sign that old habits are getting liberated, that we are moving closer to the natural open state." Eventually, we each reach a time or place where the boundaries of our comfort zone shift, allowing us a broader awareness of those previously unconscious things. Or as my friend Tom Verner says, "We choose to hunt what has been hunting us." In this way we begin to also broaden our awareness of the presence of embodied consciousness.

Even so, there is an unfortunate cloud of assumed inadequacy that hovers around the term "*un*consciousness" – a notion that we are somehow 'less than' because we are not able or willing to be fully conscious. We share, I think, a tendency to be hard on ourselves for not knowing it all.

Another Perspective

A Yogic view of the unconscious is that, in addition to the information of individual experience, it includes everything now forgotten that was once collectively known, such as the reason why that first heart beat of life occurs. From this perspective, my unconscious contains even more than the material I have chosen to repress on my own behalf and the archetypal imagery of the human collective unconscious. It (my body) also possesses the knowledge of an embodied world soul – consciousness, itself.

CHAPTER 4
LIFE AS A FOCAL POINT

Well, darkness has a hunger that's insatiable,
and lightness has a call that's hard to hear.
— The Indigo Girls (lyrics in *Closer to Fine*)

Exploring and Excavating

To come together again,
he (the average person) has to heal the dualism of his person,
of his thinking, and of his language.
— Frederick Perls

The link between the personal unconscious and the knowledge of essence was explored in depth by Carl Jung. He suggested the authentic self was the "totality of everything in the psyche" including conscious material, unconscious material related to each individual's experience (personal unconscious) and what has come to be known as the "collective unconscious." The collective *unconscious* contains both the instinctual knowledge necessary for survival and the archetypal energies that wind their way through our lives in the images of our dreams, fairy tales and cultural stories. Archetypes are "universal human symbols passed in the DNA from one generation to the next, from the earliest forms of organic life to the child being born this very minute."

According to Jung, through the process of re-telling one's personal story – bringing one's personal unconscious material into consciousness with the help of universal symbols and meanings– "the contents of the collective unconscious" and ultimately the true self, emerge.

So what is the relationship between the collective unconscious and consciousness? Here is my best *attempt* at an answer. The collective unconscious draws attention to dualities: male/female, heaven/earth, old/young, etc. While consciousness by its nature is essentially non-dual, it seems that we come to understand it by exploring the tensions created between the polarities of duality. Perhaps, in order to exist, consciousness must create and then hold together the phenomenon which we recognize as two sides of the one thing.

The central paradox of human life is that we are both unique and the same as others. On the plane of dualities, we become intimate with separateness and make judgments. Because dualities exist throughout the human experience, we have the opportunity to know something about the one thing (consciousness), which always presents itself as two.

Our innate essence is remembered as we excavate the materials of our personal unconscious and play with the tensions and metaphors of the collective unconscious. However, because the prefix "*un*" presumes the meanings "not, lack of or opposite of," the phrase "collective unconscious" unfortunately takes on a sort of negativity. I sometimes wonder, might we call it the 'collective *conscious*'?

Challenged to a Dual

An interesting phenomenon with the duality pair of consciousness and unconsciousness is that at any given moment a certain thing can be considered unconscious, and in the very next moment that same thing can become conscious and vice-versa. If we have chosen to view being conscious as more positive and being unconscious as more negative, as awareness shifts, so does our judgment of the two sides. Positive switches to negative or negative becomes positive. Kurt Goldstein writes, "They (consciousness and unconsciousness) may sometimes appear as separate entities because one or the other aspect of the total behavior is, at any given time, in the foreground as figure, while the others form the background."

Whenever there are two sides of a thing there is the automatic tendency to choose in favor of one side over the other. The root of human suffering is in such a choice. Through suffering we may discover a more complete perspective. While the choices for one side or the other of any duality remains possible, there is also a choice to sit back and remember the one thing that is created through the existence of the two sides.

Exercise

To better understand the concepts of duality and choice, imagine this: You are suddenly very small, only about 1/8 of an inch tall. You are standing on top of a table where someone has been able to place a coin (the size of a quarter) on its edge, upright and perfectly balanced. You are standing so you are facing one full round side of the coin. From this perspective, recognize the coin as "love." Say, "Ah, yes, I know love." Remember everything you know about the different kinds of love, and feel what love is like in your body.

Begin to wonder what is on the other side of this coin. Imagine you can walk around to take a look. From your new perspective see "hate" and say, "Oh, yes, I know hate." Remember all you know about hate, and feel what hate feels like in your body. Being the curious little person you are, walk around and around the coin experiencing love and hate . . . love and hate . . . and begin to choose one side of the coin as the best side to be on. Having added up your assumptions and judgments about love and hate, and just as you are about to move around to your favored side, an interesting thing will happen. About half way around, imagine a stone in your shoe, and you have to stop, sit down and shake it out. After succeeding, stand back up and realize that you are now looking straight on at the very narrow edge of the coin. From this perspective there is no love and no hate. You can't see either of them anymore, although you know both sides are still there. Look at the space between these two things. See how one supports the other, how one is known because of the existence of the other, and the two together make the one thing. There can be comfort in knowing you can choose and also of not having to choose. You can rest amidst the paradoxical understanding, that through the diversity of polarities all is one. In choosing one side, you might have forgotten what you were seeing all along was a coin.

Stephen Cope writes, "All of Yoga practice is about getting under the moment of reactivity, the moment when, in order to remain comfortable, we choose for or against one side or the other of the pairs of opposites. When the reactivity happens, as it surely will, we simply examine it in the light of the witness [Being Consciousness]."

Knowing, Thinking and Mind

Mind, like space, has no foundation.
It is not a palpable or solid thing, and it does not do anything.
Rather, the mind is a sign of a specific focal setting
being taken on Great Space (Consciousness).
— Tarthang Tulku

Thought cannot exist without consciousness,
but consciousness does not need thought.
— Eckhart Tolle

Aspects of consciousness are connected to the concepts of memory and learning. Once memory is remembered, we must learn to integrate its material into our ways of being in the world. As we consider memory, we consider mind and thought. The caution I wish to present is this: It is important to move away from speaking as if mind and thought exist somewhere separately from the body as Descartes once suggested. Certainly Candice Pert's research indicates this is not the case.

Continuing to separate the concepts of being conscious from being unconscious perpetuates a further splitting of mind from body. Keeping the concept that "all is embodied," it *could* be said that both conscious and unconscious material exists on a simple spectrum of available awareness of sensation, thought, emotion and divine essence. All information is inside, waiting for awareness to occur.

Some information is known through cognitive thought. Some is known without thinking through felt experience.

Awareness is the Thing

With respect to self-understanding, what is perhaps most valuable to experience is the ongoing dance between the qualities and quantities of awareness. Awareness happens through the body. If we are prisms or focal points for one consciousness who have for any number of individual and collective reasons forgotten that we are this, then the spectrum of awareness ranges from "I am unaware" all the way to "I am awareness itself."

I wrote the following poem about one year after my Long Trail journey. I wrote it during transition from summer to fall, from unaware to awareness.

Momentary Crossing

> *There are times when,*
> *If the circumstances are just right,*
> *Like a full moon,*
> *A light rain,*
> *Twilight, or fog,*
> *There is a momentary crossing*
> *From time to timelessness,*
> *Form to Formless,*
> *Blood and bone to earth and rock,*
> *Past and future to present.*
>
> *Where the atoms, the molecules of me*
> *Forget to stop*
> *From fusing into the earth and other places*
> *Where I am not lost, but found,*
> *Not part, but whole,*
> *No longer longing for myself.*

Because we are human right now, we are either aware or unaware. Because we are consciousness always, we are awareness itself. The constant flow of shifting awareness between being human and being divine can be felt in the body. We are both the watcher and the watched, the still point and the dance. We live our own human drama while developing a sense of our own dharma (purpose) in relation to the flow of all life. Stephen Cope writes, "Beneath the surface of our separation, we feel the hidden, unseen threads that link us."

To me existence *does* feels like an ebb and flow; sometimes there are waves that roll toward the shore of my uniqueness and other times the tides of my true essence rise up. And neither one destroys the other. Each is validated.

A Wheel of a Continuum

We are a circle within a circle . . . With no beginning and never ending.
— Rick Hamouris (lyrics from *Welcome to Annwfn*)

If we were to look at ourselves in relation to consciousness on a continuum of awareness, it might resemble the wheel-like rendition on the following page.

This model is intended to represent awareness as a flow. We are continually moving in or out of each area on the continuum. We are even, sometimes, in more than one area at the same time, though one or the other is somehow more present at any given moment. Through the figure/ground flow of what we can feel in our bodies, we move across the continuum of our awareness. When we are awake in the world of direct sensation and experience, and even when we are asleep and dreaming, we experience the consciousness that we essentially are as well as our unique human representation of that consciousness as *interplay*. Pema Chödrön writes, "We are all a paradoxical bundle of rich potential that consists of both neurosis and wisdom."

"I am awareness, itself."

"I am aware that I might be awareness, itself."

"I am unaware."

Consciousness

"I am aware of awareness."

"I am aware of how I need to cope right now. I repress what I need to in order to cope successfully."

"I find it difficult to be aware in the midst of my life situations and I suppress many things in an unhealthy way."

"I intend to become more aware in the midst of my life situations and I sometimes need to suppress my feelings in a healthy way."

Meditation

Use you imagination and your body sensations to create a deeper understanding of the continuum of awareness. In seated meditation, feel your body as if it were a droplet of rain water that has fallen from the sky in slow motion and has just touched down on the surface of the ground. The bottom part of the droplet – of you – is spreading out in all directions, making a widening droplet base while the upper part of you (of the droplet) is still somewhat suspended from above , peaked, as if it were still falling from the sky. You are spreading out at the bottom, grounded, and at the same time lifting up at the top. Between these upper and lower areas, you can discover a sense of an intrinsic, buoyant energy – a tension arc of awareness.

Now imagine that some of the water in you, in the droplet, is clear enough to see through, while other areas have varying degrees of cloudiness. Some of your water is murky with unknown particles flowing around in it, and some is muddy, thick and inexplicable. Notice the different degrees of clarity in this water droplet – in your body – and remember that your are really one droplet, one you.

Exhale and invite some of the cloudier areas to settle out a bit, waiting to receive information in whatever way it wants to come, as thought, emotion, image, memory or more sensation.

Turn your focus to the entirety of the water droplet . . .the entirety of your body. Breathe, allowing yourself to finish dropping. Notice what it is like to let go of your edges a little bit, or a lot – to melt your boundaries for just a few seconds, as if you were water finally oozing out into the ground. Watch for any momentary tiny moments of union with something else while not losing yourself. As these moments come, get a sense of what that is like. A peaceful letting go? A greater lightness? See that as a droplet, unique with your own degrees of clarity and murkiness, you remain essentially water.

Shifting

Although stillness and silence can enhance awareness, awareness itself is not a still thing. Its nature is to circle and spiral, to be seen and unseen, to focus in and fade away as it moves us toward change. Sometimes it jumps up large while other times it presents itself so subtly that we hardly notice we have accomplished something on our own behalf.

Awareness can shift even at the "I am unaware" level. Unconscious material moves across the continuum to a new place. Writer Alice Walker spoke beautifully to this when she wrote, "Perhaps my unconscious begins working on poems from these emotions (ones she would like to explore) long before I am aware of it." I have noticed these kinds of shifts occurring as I sleep. I wake up with new insights and answers to problems.

A continuum perspective such as the one presented above supports my notion that awareness is sometimes figure and sometimes ground. As in the droplet image, some things stand out clearly from the murky background while others, at times, do not.

Broadening Views

From my journal, January 21, 2002 (after Yoga practice):

Today, while driving home, I realized that I am beginning to look past the houses as I drive by them, into the backyards, and I'm wondering about the woods and fields and hills behind them – how they connect, where they go . . . what's out there? This is new for me. Could it be that I am beginning to look 'past the surface'? I feel a growing curiosity to explore and less fear of doing so. More of the time, I know I won't get lost.

Not being, at the time, efficient and accurate with a map or compass, it was my wise choice to stay on the well-worn trail when I was hiking across Vermont. It would not have been the best idea for me to bushwhack through unknown, unpredictable territory without preparation. This is also true as one begins a sincere journey of self-discovery. It felt safer to start small, moving one step at a time into what was already partially known. Later on, as my ability to be my body – to enlist both map and compass – improved, the off-trail ground became enticingly more interesting and secure.

To Repress or to Suppress?

In the wheel model of awareness I used the words "suppress" and "repress." I attribute no judgment of right or wrong, better or best, to either of these strategies for getting along in the world.

Suppression happens when we hold back emotions, thoughts, beliefs, sensations and actions in association with our present situation. We choose against a full or even a partial expression of our experience for various reasons, such as worry over social unacceptability, desire to follow the crowd, wishes to protect the feelings of another, fears of non-acceptance and self-devaluation. We often mistake this type of suppression for a positive attitude; we suck it up in order to plow through the situation at hand.

In a *healthy* suppression situation, we are aware of our present emotions and thoughts, as well as the connected sensations in our bodies, even though we choose not to act them out. We understand at some point we need to find ways of appropriate expression, and we do. Sometimes we are simply aware of being uncomfortable. We know something is not quite right, but in the heat of the moment we are not fully aware of what is wrong. If we choose to take the time to acknowledge our healthy suppressions, addressing related body sensations and letting go of present control, we can usually discover how to make life adjustments that can turn our suppression into expression . . . or how to express what was suppressed. We can change our relationship to our situations and move one step closer to self-understanding in the process.

Unhealthy suppression, on the other hand, offers us bigger challenges and also wider opportunities for learning about oneself. This is really just a more intensified version of healthy suppression. In this version, we give up the possibility of self-expression in a self-sacrificing manner. We find ways to ignore the messages from our bodies, losing sight of the value of emotional expression. We deny sadness, fear, anxiety, anger and opinion, believing them to be useless in the face of our life circumstances. We may still possess a low level of awareness that something is unbalanced, yet any deeper investigation is also denied.

Even though one's body might be reacting strongly due to the stress of unhealthy suppression, it is sometimes possible to lose all sense of corresponding emotions. Feelings become what Lydia Temoshok refers to as "phantom emotions." When asked about an emotion such as anger, an individual understands anger but is unable to allow or to recognize this feeling occurring in him or herself.

The material of unhealthy suppression may eventually lead to related symptoms or conditions. Chronic discomforts or pain may develop over time and later intensify. We work hard to "keep things in," imagining the results and in a progressive attempt to draw awareness to phantom emotions, of letting them out to be harder still.

Unhealthy suppression also appears to be intimately connected to our immune system's strength. Temoshok's research in this area reveals that not only does suppressing thoughts, emotions and sensations in this way cloud authenticity, but it also inhibits our immune system's ability to keep us well.

Repression is the term given to an automatic blocking of the memory of experience from awareness. It is the *"I am unaware"* point on the wheel continuum. For positive reasons, we have refused to permit the existence of certain events as well as associated emotions and sensations. We lower a thick veil over those things that are far too difficult to know in an attempt to function as best we can, and remain unaware that repression is occurring. Psychotherapist, Fritz Perls, explains, "In repression . . . we have lost awareness both of what is repressed and the process by which we do the repressing."

Repression can be called "the motivated forgetting of the disagreeable." Motivated forgetting is difficult work, too. The doing of repression lends a whole new meaning to the notion of "working overtime." The thickness of the veil must be maintained. All we may be aware of is the fatigue associated with the effort of repression.

However, my own experience of repression has included similar and somewhat different qualities. While I repressed, for many years, some aspects of my past, I did maintain (as with suppression) a lingering sense that something was trying to be known. In other words, I was not oblivious to a need for some sort of expression. As a child

I was repeatedly ill. Most of my ailments were related to my throat and lungs, the parts of my body most involved with expression. I was also plagued with allergic reactions, which I feel were reflective of the anxiety connected to my abuse and the way my skin was touched.

In my earlier days of receiving psychotherapy, repressed material began to move forward into my awareness. Later, as I investigated my body more and more through Yoga, remaining elements of memory gradually and safely rose to the surface. I remembered as I was ready to do so. As I reflect on both therapeutic experiences, I realize that although I appreciated the assistance of talk therapy, I felt pushed rather than drawn to explore my history. I also found it easy to creatively sidestep my way through many sessions by ignoring body sensations, putting on a good face and pretending things were other than they actually were. Without my body's involvement, I could remain neutral. My mind was less truthful than my body.

Yoga and Yoga Therapy, which fully involved my body (me) in my process, curiously drew me in the direction of repressed memory one sensation at a time. The process was not comfortable, but it was safe and non-invasive. There were no externally imposed expectations as I had imagined were present in psychotherapy . . . no efforts to "fix me," either from the outside in, or from the inside out. Through connecting the dots of sensation, emotion, thought and essence I gradually found my own way.

A Recent Release

Not long ago I was able to recall some lingering repressed information. I am not a small woman. I am average in height and weight, but I always have felt too big. My sensations of always being too big hung around me at every turn, yet I avoided wondering about the reasons why this perception of myself persisted. I married a man who is smaller than me. All of my daughters are much smaller than me, so at family gatherings I felt as if I loomed large – somehow too there, too conspicuous – too present.

As my practice of Yoga became a larger part of my life, this sensation of being too big grew to the point where I could no longer deny that there was some great importance to my sensations. I began to ask why I was too big, when I really wasn't. What did the feeling of bigness have to do with me? Each Yoga practice brought me further to the edge of something, some answer to my question that would just about break through, but not quite.

After a week of particularly intense practice, my husband David and I had a chance to get away for a romantic break. During an intimate interlude, the dam I had built against my body's efforts to tell me my truth finally broke. I began to sob, my whole just the right size body shuddering with remembering.

My body matured at an early age. I was taller than most by the time I was nine and filled out into a woman's shape before I was ten. I appeared much older than I really was. This trait drew the sexual abusers of my family – both male and female – in my direction. For forty years, I had been blaming myself for being too big, accepting responsibility that was not mine, holding in my cells, tormented by my bigness every day. David held me, while I screamed, wailed and emptied my body of the bigness and the shame that was stuck inside it.

I am not as big anymore, definitely not too big. But every now and then I get that large sense for a moment, pay it some acknowledgement, and it fades away.

Suppressed and repressed information is innocently held in our cells and tissues, perhaps most widely within our muscles and fascia. The continued choice to control emotion and experience may eventually lead to reduced or even lost proprioception over those areas of the body that are holding those memories, stories, thoughts and feelings. However, awareness can shift when the timing is right. In the meantime, while we might remain unready to bring material into awareness or into expression, our bodies will begin to reflect what is being held inside through sensation. Turning awareness toward sensation, we can begin the process of remembering.

Chapter 5

Becoming Self-ish

What we are looking for is what is looking.
— St. Francis of Assisi

When one can hear the voice of the Self and learn to obey it,
one walks and talks with authenticity.
— Connie Zweig and Steve Wolf

Dressed in Layers

From a dream I had on day two of a Yoga Therapy intensive:

I am standing dressed in layers of clothing. I am wondering who dressed me like this – in layers. An old woman accompanies me. She and someone else try to pull a vest off over my head – after I've asked them to. But I say, 'No, I can do it myself. I can undo the zipper.'

Although we are gifted with a variety of teachers and mentors along the paths of self-revelation, in the end it is ourselves who remove the layers of belief that cover up who we truly are. I have spent a great deal of time considering the self-beliefs that prevent me from moving more fully into life. My "I am too big" belief is one example. On the mat in Yoga postures and in meditation, I have proclaimed my limiting judgments out loud, heightening my awareness of each one and watching how each affects my body.

One day, early on in my Yoga journey, I actually counted the layers of my beliefs. At the time, there were seven of them: 1) I'm too big. 2) I'm not good enough. 3) I'm not pretty enough. 4) I'm not interesting enough. 5) I'm a victim. 6) I'm invisible. 7) Falling down will kill me.

I then found an article of clothing to represent each belief. As I put on each garment, I spoke the belief that it represented. Once they are all in place, I stood dressed in my layers.

From this perspective, my layers were exaggerated and heavily tangible. It was frustrating to realize I had dressed myself this way. I was also a little angry with myself. I hung around for a while in my layers, allowing the frustration of this to land in me. I felt it gather in my shoulders, upper back and neck. No wonder there was so much tension there. I began to get claustrophobic. I wondered how many layers I would need to remove in order to feel just right.

I stood very still, which was not easy. I wanted to move around enough to distract myself from the sensation of the layers. As I stood, however, I was able to contact a more real me waiting beneath all the layers. The layers were representative of my real life experience, but they were like masks I had forced myself to wear. There was something more to me than these limitations. I could feel the untruth in each one. Underneath, my more real self – the core part of me that knew without thinking held no judgment against the added layers, just a curiosity about them and a sincere interest in letting them go.

Slowly, almost ceremoniously, I removed each garment layer. I remembered to acknowledge the truth that each one had once served a necessary purpose of some sort. I also announced the removal of each belief, pausing to notice what was happening in my body as I did so. I felt myself grow lighter, cooler and free. At the same time, I felt sensations of vulnerability, a nakedness that I was not completely ready for. I did, however, get a sense of what might lie ahead should I choose to do some letting go, and I could begin to imagine which beliefs might be the easiest to shed.

Exercise

Take a few minutes and consider any beliefs you hold about yourself that stand in your way as you move through life. My "I am too big" belief is an example of this type of limiting belief. Write them down in your journal. Next, while either standing or sitting quietly, say each one out loud to yourself. It may help to close your eyes as you say the words. Each time you announce one of your beliefs, notice what is happening in your body. You may find that you need to speak the words more than once in order to heighten your awareness. Write down any body experiences that occur in your journal next to the corresponding belief. Now, count up your layers of beliefs and find an article of clothing that can represent each one. As you put on each garment, speak the belief that it represents. Once they are all on, stand dressed in your layers. What's happening now? What's not happening? It's important that you consider your own answer to this question before reading on.

From this perspective, layers seem very real. Who dressed you this way? Do you have a sense that there is a *you* within the layers that is somehow more authentic? Make some sort of contact with this more real aspect of you. If you are not sure about how to do this, imagine what it would be like to have a more real layer. Where in your body do you feel this kind of realness?

Slowly, ceremoniously, remove each garment layer. Announce the removal of each belief, pausing to notice what's happening in your body when you do this. Take some time to write about this experience in your journal.

Aspects of Self

The individual self that we long to know is, at its essence, a focal point of one consciousness, which is embodied in all things. As it inhabits us, consciousness, in yogic philosophy, is called Jivatman, the "living self" or "individuated consciousness." Jivatman is considered the individual manifestation of Atman, the entire field of human consciousness. Expanding farther, Atman is the human field representation of Brahman, the vast expanse of "that which grows and causes everything to grow." Whatever one might choose to label these layers of a unitary consciousness, it was such a vastness that I sensed as the somehow more real aspect of myself, underneath the layers of my limiting beliefs. It is this essence that we recognize through being in a body when we are present to everyday miracles. I often wonder how my life might be different if I could consistently remember I am, (my body is), one such miracle.

Our cells contain the knowledge of our divinity as well as the history and current events of our humanness. We are inherent wisdom, personal story and collective information simultaneously. Our wisdom lies within the abiding presence of cellular consciousness, while our stories lie in our genetic, cellular memory. All is embodied! If this isn't a miracle, I don't know what is!

However, while it is important to remember the essential reality that we are divine, it is equally important to gain an understanding of the individual aspects of our personal stories. It is by doing the latter, by emptying out the backpack, that we remember the richness of our authenticity. The exploration of individuality provides us with the opportunity to reveal Jivatman (and ultimately Atman and Brahman). The divine cannot be known without the human and vise-versa. Awareness of one brings awareness of the other.

Even as I feel the truth of this resonating in my body, in the core of me, it also seems as if I am made up of many selves, each with their own dharma and agendas. I frequently catch myself saying, "There is a part of me that . . . . and another part of me that. . . ."

I believe that it is part of the human experience to exist in a state of healthy multiplicity. These seemingly separate selves offer rotational leadership given our life situation. I have many: the victim, the warrior, the comforter, the quitter, the thinker, the judge, the jury, and the child, to name a few. Each has played a valuable role. Each contributes to my particular expression of the consciousness that I am.

Contemporary psychotherapist, Richard Swartz, refers to these aspects of individual self as our internal family system. He recognizes the many parts or sub-personalities that feel like "separate internal people of different ages, talents and temperaments" who seem to inhabit us in an interactive or argumentative manner. These parts, who wish to play productive roles (and do so most of the time), can get carried away and become destructive. The key is to arrive at a consensus of parts where all are integrated through the common goal of creating balance. As integration occurs, the din of the internal conversations quiets and the wisdom of the self can be heard again.

Parts such as these are related to ego and the survival of our humanness. Ego is the personal strategy through which we know our separateness – our I-ness. It is stubborn and vulnerable, has a flair for drama, and gets entangled in thoughts and strategies. It is past, future and survival oriented. Ego loves the arguments and judgments of dualities, and identifies with status, appearance and possessions. Ego parts want to know the facts and are uncomfortable with vague subtleties such as the concept of an authentic self. They tend to assume there is generally something wrong with us and something wrong with the world, hence they create problems for their own amusement.

"It is the ego that deludes itself that there are two selves, one of which we are conscious now, the person, and the other, the Divine, of which we will one day be conscious. This is false. There is only one Self and it is fully conscious now and ever," wrote Maharshi.

When our awareness is focused on our I-ness, we forget our universal nature and risk remaining stuck in our separateness. While the ego tends to resist knowing the authentic self for fear of getting lost in the process of a non-separate awareness, all it really wants is recognition for an important job well done.

Still, a strong ego is a valuable asset. It is likely that a strong sense of I-ness supports our ability to listen to the language of the body and ask tough questions about one's stories. Through ego we discern what is valuable to us on our chosen paths, and what can be left behind us as compost for something better. If not for ego, we would not know separateness. Without experiencing separateness, can we remember union?

Developmentalists suggest that we spend a great deal of our lives alternating between the yearning to be separate or different from the rest and a desire to be the same as or included with the rest. We practice being each way until we step around the coin and gain the perspective that we are both. We allow equal room for both inhabitants.

Our ego, I-ness and uniqueness do not have to step aside in order for our authenticity to be revealed. In fact, paradoxically, through our recognition of oneness, ego and uniqueness become richer and stronger. The self that is felt at the core of the body beneath all the layers of personal information becomes counsel and guide for the helpful ego.

Robert and the Horse

The following is a recent example of a conversation between an ego and the resulting wise counsel from my larger self part. It arose during a standing meditation and a Phoenix Rising Yoga Therapy process known as Two-Part Dialogue.

My open place was my belly. It felt calm and full of room (grounded). It felt like a cradle or a hammock. I brought it even more present by rocking back and forth. I remembered another time, when I had felt this way, was when I was rocking my baby. I began to weep remembering that I was so young when Jenny was born. I knew how to mother her from this open place, but I also still needed mothering myself. I had been very confused and unsure of my mothering ability in my mind, but this place had instinctively known what to do. I named this place "Cradle."

My restricted place was my right knee (the one that had wanted to run away at other times). My right thigh was pulling up and my knee wanted to lock back. I exaggerated this by contracting my thigh and allowing the locking to occur, which made my whole body start to subtly shake. This place was "Stubborn." I remembered a cornucopia of times, when I resisted so many things with my stubbornness, including both mothering and allowing myself to be nurtured. Stubborn was an uncomfortable, yet very familiar place, while Cradle was more comfortable and less familiar.

When Stubborn spoke to Cradle, it was with the voice of a little girl, who sang "Na na na-na-na. You can't make me!" When Cradle spoke to Stubborn, she offered that she was just going to 'be' there no matter what, and stubborn could come to her or not. Either way was okay with Cradle, because Cradle was simply there with no agenda.

Stubborn replied, "You say that now, but I don't believe you. If I come, you might go away – abandon me." Cradle replied she could not or would not try to change Stubborn's mind about that. She just was going to be there doing her cradle thing.

As the conversation went on, I remembered a scene from the film The Horse Whisperer, in which the main character played by Robert Redford is trying to re-ground a spirited horse that has been severely traumatized. In the scene I was remembering, the horse has gotten loose and is running in circles in a large field, not willing to be caught. Robert Redford simply sits down in the center of the field and stays there all day. By dusk the horse's curiosity has gotten the better of him, and he has moved in close enough to touch the man. Eventually they walk quietly together back to the barn, the horse's fears and stubbornness quieted.

The situation occurring between my belly and my leg felt like this scene in the movie: Cradle calmly waiting, understanding both herself and Stubborn, not trying to make anything happen. Stubborn, starting to circle, is still resistant to but curious about Cradle.

I renamed my parts, calling my belly area Robert and my knee Horse.

Then the wisdom from self came through, "Be still and wait." As I spoke them, the ground shifted. "Be still and wait!" I have been chasing spooked horses – my husband, my daughter, my thesis and myself. I have not been reaching out from this grounded place. But I can because I know it is there. How simple. Be still and wait for the horse to come in, for Jenny to come closer, for David to trust my process, for my thesis to unfold, for me to know myself. Be still and wait for the ground to shift, re-ground myself and reach out again. Be still and wait. Be still and wait.

Throughout my practice of body awareness I have spoken with many such parts, leaders and followers, such as the victim, the hero, the child, the stubborn one and the protector. There were also parts whose existence I did not want to admit, such as the angry, fierce part. Most importantly, by experiencing these aspects of my individuality in my body, I am less pushed through life by my phantom parts. I am more guided by my authentic self. By bringing each part into the light of awareness and acknowledging its worth and appreciating the role each part plays, I began to remember my true realness. I have found this process to be as Cope describes: "The witness emerges naturally when we have developed a good enough sense of the ego self."

The authentic self that I am discovering, through experiencing my body, is the subtlest part of me that is never unconscious. It is the 'part' of me that is abiding wisdom – the one who knows without thinking. Self is the compassionate, non-judgmental witness that simplifies and unifies all things – the "transpersonal voice" within the "personal life."

I have come to recognize self in the space between the dualities of my human existence. She is the space between my in breath and my out breath – the still point. Self is a collective voice of wisdom that also speaks for me. It is the part of me that I truly am. I am inherent understanding. I am my own guru, my own agent of change, my own fairy godmother, whether I remember this 24/7 or not.

Robert Kegan suggested that we can best be understood as "an ever progressive motion engaged in giving itself a new form." I propose that instead we are "ever progressive, non-linear, spiraling energies engaged in revealing who we already are." Our process is to flow between the understanding of our separate uniqueness and our unified oneness. I-ness and self weave a web of wisdom and information throughout our bodies embedded in our connective fascial tissue and other body systems. As does everything in the universe, we "exist in a state of potentiality, which already contains the finished product within it." Everything is already okay, even all of those interesting or scary parts. As Cope has said, we are "fully in the dance and, at the same time, . . . fully in the calmly abiding center."

Yogi Amrit Desai summarizes my attempts at explaining the emerging self through the process of Yoga. He said, "In Yoga, there is only one problem and one solution: The problem is that we've forgotten who we are; the solution is to remember who we are, to reidentify with the entire reality of Atman."

The experience of being *human* is a multi-faceted, embodied process. It is the thrilling whirlwind of a hurricane. The experience of being *consciousness* (divine) is a centering, grounding, single-faceted phenomenon that is also embodied. It is the calm, abiding eye of the hurricane.

Through a greater awareness and understanding of the sensations and qualities of both the whirlwind *and* the eye, I come to know my authenticity. I am both.

Tantra Yoga (often associated with Kundalini Yoga) represents a dimension of Hinduism that emphasizes personal embodied experience and experimentation. Masters of Tantra distinguish between the worldly (human) level of reality and the wisdom-informed, ultimate level of reality. The worldly reality is shifting and somewhat unreliable, full of possible illusions and assumptions, but practical for negotiating life. The informed reality is reliable in its wisdom, but unpractical within the world without a body. The union of the two is the self. In the embodied state, inherent wisdom finds balance with the worldly level of reality.

The ideal of Tantra Yoga is "to live in the world out of the fullness of Self-realization rather than to withdraw from life in order to gain enlightenment." Yet classical Yoga also offers the perspective that it is possible, even desirable, to "traverse the different levels of existence until, at the moment of liberation, . . . [one can] leave the orbit of Nature altogether." So, it seems as if choice is at the crux of a Yogic journey. Either we embrace embodiment as the way to self-realization or we spend our lives preparing to transcend it. Did we come here to live life fully, or did we come to separate from it?

For me, the key is to walk comfortably in both the world of human experience and the world of divine grace – to understand and value all that I embody. This is the aim of *my* Yoga: To arrive at this balance of living matter and unifying energy. My intention is not to transcend my body, but to live more fully in it. Throughout my process, my thoughts, emotions, attitudes and beliefs may change, but the wisdom-informed reality of me will not.

Fellow hiker, Connie Batten, in the collections of essays in *Being Bodies: Buddhist Women on the Paradox of Embodiment*, writes, "If I am one of the prisms through which the universe perceives itself, it is part of my purpose to maintain a distinct and separate position made up of personal history, desire for safety, and fear of extinction. And as a temporary bubble afloat on the stream of universal flux, I am sometimes given the gift of knowing in utter effortlessness that there are also no distinctions."

Even though the life work of many dedicated and respected individuals leads us toward definitions of such things as consciousness and self, there are, as yet, no exact answers. When it comes to aspects of being, there are many gaps of understanding between the layers of subjective experience and objective observation.

I remain confident that the future will bring us back to embodiment and direct experience as the key elements of understanding self, relationship and purpose. In the meantime, each of us can work in this direction in personal and collective ways. By turning inward to our own experience we learn about our own authenticity. By knowing who we essentially are, we soften our ways of being in the world, inviting others to do the same through our example.

Part Two:

Building on the Foundation

CHAPTER 6
"FEELING" REAL

I wish I could show you,
When you are lonely or in darkness,
The Astonishing Light
Of your own Being!

— Hafiz

One is ready to know what is.
One is not interested in what can be,
what should be, what ought to be . . .
one is interested only in that which is,
because only the real can free you,
only the reality can become liberation.

— Bhagwan S. Rajneesh

From a letter I wrote in the spring of 2003:

Yes, something important is taking place in me. Am I sure what it is? Well, I know it is safe and perfectly timed. I ask, as I am ready to listen, and I receive what I ask for. I never expected that shifts in awareness would be comfortable, but they are not as painful as the pain of remaining the same as before. Psychotherapy has played an earlier important role in my life but stopped short of creating clarity around authenticity. Where psychotherapy left off, Yoga and Yoga Therapy began to provide such clarity. I have not and do not seek disembodiment or escape. Quite the opposite, I somehow feel more real in my body – with that "different center of gravity" that you mention in your letter. As Margery Williams

writes in The Velveteen Rabbit: *"Real isn't how you are made,"*
said the Skin Horse. "It's a thing that happens to you." "Does it
hurt?" asked the Rabbit. "Sometimes," said the Skin Horse, for
he was always truthful.

Moving Toward Self

A focus of Yoga is to change one's awareness of oneself and one's
relationship to the world. Awareness begins by awakening to the
felt realness of one's body, the personal information it holds and the
essence of self that it is. Awakening begins with a quickening – a body
sensation that invites curiosity and a sort of animation toward change.
Quickening is the feeling that throws a spark that has the potential to
light the fire of transformation.

Quickening

When your secret heart cannot speak so easily, come on darlin',
  from a whisper start – to have a little faith in me.
  — Van Morrison (lyrics from *Have a Little Faith in Me*)

My first recognition of quickening in my own body was the
instant when my baby, Jennifer, first flickered within my womb. It was
a startling sense of energy moving inside me, and it was absolutely
one of those everyday miracles when I instantly, but only for a few
seconds, recognized the vastness of my being. I was nineteen years
old, still adding layers and not at all ready to consider my authenticity.
Each day was already way too real. Yet, here I am thirty-five years
later, remembering and even feeling that first quickening sensation in
my body, realizing now how that experience gave rise to my ability to
recognize the quickening moments yet to come. Far less subtle than
the experiences I would notice later in my life, this moment remains
in me as strong as it was back then.

Most moments of quickening are not as strong. Rather these
moments appear in many forms, all of them sensationally similar.
While the fetal quickening of pregnancy announces that something is
right with how things are, this is not always the case. While this first

sensation had been acutely specific in my womb, most quickening sensations are body wide across the total flow of neuropeptides.

We could go back to the image of the princess and the pea. Through all the layers of mattresses, she knew something was not quite right with the way things were. This is often the sense with quickening; there is a tiny, but growing, dissatisfaction with something that calls us to pay attention.

Often there is a slight and uniquely edgy quality to quickening that can easily be overlooked. Depending on our readiness to explore what might be beneath these body cues, we might decide either to focus awareness on it or to suppress both the sensation and our curiosity. However we decide, the body persists, and quickening can become as Tolle describes, "background static" waiting for us to tune into the important messages that are arising.

A much more subtle experience with quickening occurred when I was nearing the end of my Phoenix Rising Yoga Therapy training. I was feeling generally restless. My body was squirmy, and I was having trouble focusing on finishing the required work for graduation. It was one of those quickenings which I could have chosen to push aside or push through. But I recognized there was probably something important about these sensations and called a fellow practitioner to schedule a much needed Yoga Therapy session for myself.

I think that quickening is a function of the self, what Eugene Gendlin called a "felt sense." In Yogic terms, quickening is the feeling of the "inborn seed of consciousness" cracking open inside us, its sprouting roots tickling our heart's attention.

This tickling is a gentle invitation to come closer to lifting the veils we have draped over the parts of us that we have not wanted to see. It becomes as if the self messes up the veil, turning it askew, so that a certain aspect of us begins to stick out. We then have two choices. We can become irritated, in which case we rush to put the veil back in place, or we can sit with the edginess of the 'material' until we are willing to at least acknowledge such a part of us exists.

When we are noticing a quickening in our bodies, a fluttering of curiosity, a subtle cross cell anxiety, we benefit by realizing what we are noticing is a divine invitation to act on our own behalf. We are receiving an opportunity to explore the parts of us we are ready to know and understand, including our authentic centers. In this way quickening is loaded with the potential for heightened self-awareness and personal change.

The body provides a safe way into the places that have seemed risky to visit. Whatever is ready to happen probably will happen, if we are brave enough to open the body's invitation. Our human tendency is to fear what is already in us, but body and self would not offer us the invitations of quickening, if we (our ego natured parts) were not somehow ready to RSVP affirmatively. Yet, an act of courage is often necessary in order to take the risk of learning the mystery behind the quickening. As Jack Kornfield writes, ". . . .the unknown territory of initiation will open before us only to the extent that we turn our whole being courageously toward it."

Creating Space

From my journal, April 2002:

> *Fish posture brings up the same thing that my earlier massage did. For some reason my left calf was urging me to do something, and when I asked it what it wanted me to do, it told me I needed to have a lawn sale! 'Do spring cleaning! Uncover the walls that you keep stumbling over! Get rid of the clutter! At least do it metaphorically by cleaning out your house. Give up some things you're attached to. Get the point?'*
>
> *Fish is telling me the same thing – 'Make room to receive love! Start on a stuff removal ritual of physical objects and remain aware of the importance of what you are doing.' I realize that I must pay special attention to the stuff in the upstairs in the least seen rooms!*

My practices of Yoga and Yoga Therapy have become my ways of turning toward the quickening sensation of my body with trust and receptivity. The postures and meditations that I include provide me with the foundational space in which I can gain much clearer perspectives of myself. The space I am referring to is the space of my body – a space for self. For change to occur, it is essential to create within myself an open, un-layered space. This process requires a willingness to allow for the possibility that I already know who I am and what is best for me. And I must be ready to open to this possibility with a degree of self-compassion and non-judgment.

Creating space for the possibility of self is both the simplest and the hardest thing we could do. It is simple because it requires only a letting go of all those things that we hang onto in order to create our seemingly safe separateness. It is difficult for the same reason. It is as easy as taking off the backpack and as hard as walking away from everything of importance that is in it. We may be curious about the mysterious potential of quickening sensations, but we will likely need to begin to turn away from old and dear patterns of behavior in the process of satisfying that curiosity. We cannot enter the mystery without first being willing to let go of its control.

How do we become willing to relinquish enough control and be ready to enter the mystery? For me, it is whenever the pain of entering into the unknown becomes less than the pain of remaining outside.

In *Yoga and the Quest for the True Self*, Stephen Cope describes certain aspects of transformative space. While he suggests these are necessary for the creation of what we might call "externally oriented space," I would like to add they can also be considered as necessary aspects of "internally oriented space." Keep the following design elements in mind, as you prepare to turn in the direction of the felt sense of quickening.

In order to create space for receiving the messages of quickening and of moving deeper into awareness, you need:

- An attitude of acceptance. (Everything is already okay just as it is — even if it seems imperfect. We are ready and willing to become actively receptive to sensation and meaning.)

- An offer of refuge. (We will not judge ourselves. We will be self-compassionate.)

- Permission to not know. (We don't have to have the answers in order to ask the questions.)

- Consistency in relationship. (We find ways to keep the conversation with self evolving slowly through our body's language.)

- Creative experimentation. (We are open to possibilities, as we try on various ways of learning about self. We will explore many paths of discovery, day by day.)

- Opportunities to discover self through our unique experience. (Our discovery is free of rules, expectations and assumptions.)

All of the above can be seen as helpful aspects of the transformative space we can potentially create within ourselves. Creating such a space allows us to come toward truth, even as we feel our vulnerability.

I scheduled that Yoga Therapy session about quickening with a very skilled practitioner whom I had known for quite some time. I knew the transformative space she would create and hold for me would match the one I was holding for myself. As I drove to this session, I became more and more anxious about what it might entail. *The quickening was already becoming intensified through my responding to it. I found myself repeating my promises, "Acceptance . . . courage . . . opportunity. No judgment . . . compassion. Everything is already okay – even not knowing."*

It is helpful to know that the whole space does not have to open all at once. A door can be cracked open rather than swung wide. Transformative space will grow on its own as we continue to step out of its way. And at those times when it is difficult to let that whisper start or even to relate to the concept of opening up such a space, we always can just pretend we can do it. We can pretend it is possible. Pretending has an almost magical way of leading us back to truth. Within imagination hides intention. As with the Velveteen Rabbit and a little wooden fellow named Pinocchio, we become real through our intention.

Awakening and Awareness

> *Prepare to meet yourself through your body.*
> *This body . . . this moment . . . this breath.*
>   — Michael Lee

> *Look at my body. You will see the entire universe there.*
> *And all are part of the same, which is me.*
>   — from *The Bhagavad Gita*
> "Lord's Song," Yoga scripture from the third or fourth century BCE

From my journal, November 2002:

> *Emerging into her vulnerability,*
> *Sleek Heart Warrior.*
> *Her athletic grace*
> *Opens me to compassion.*
> *Soft strength holds Courage.*

Awakening and awareness begin as soon as we accept the invitation of quickening. Awakening has to do with the first glimpses of what lies behind the mysteries of quickening. Awareness has to do with the degree of attention and focus we give to our awakening knowledge. I have come to know all of this through my body. After all, where else would it possibly be?

There is a morphing, shifting, growing feeling when awakening, a cell by cell perspective of the many possible meanings of quickening. Awareness, on the other hand, requires a closer-up, yet open-minded focus, on what awakening has brought to the surface of our attention. There are, I think, four things that are necessary to enable the processes of awakening and awareness to occur: silence, breath, spontaneity and remaining present.

My Yoga Therapy session began, as always, with a meditation, the intention of which was to allow the processes of awakening and awareness to begin. As I sat on the mat in meditation position, the squirminess of my body became more apparent than ever. It was not long before I also knew the message of this now familiar quickening. My body felt full of loose ends – disconnected from each other – wiggling throughout my cells and systems. The loose ends were related to the work of learning how to become a Yoga Therapy practitioner. After six months of deep, intense exploration of the layers of me that shrouded my authentic self, there was something left undone – at loose ends.

This awakening was also present in my breath. In between, what were mostly long, full, open, relaxed breaths were some short, quick, gasping ones. These breaths were in such contrast to the longer ones that they were really getting my attention. Here is where the wider search for awakening began to evolve into more focused awareness. This shorter breathing hidden between the regular breaths was like a secret. It was the type of secret breath you would take if you were trying to be so quiet that no one would know you were there. I remember being a little surprised at this point that there was no question as to whether or not I would allow a further look into what the secret was.

My daily practice of Yoga had provided me with the strength to remain curious. My choice was to go on. My intention for this Yoga Therapy session was to as fully as possible, right now, explore the loose ends and the secret breath within the safety of the personal transformational space I had worked so hard to clear.

It makes sense to me to speak about awakening and awareness almost in the same breath. As with individual self and universal self, they cannot be separated, although they are different aspects of the one thing. Awakening invites awareness. Awareness opens the door of internal transformative space a bit wider and reciprocates by inviting new awakenings (as well as more quickenings). In the practice of Yoga and in moments of daily living, there can be a constant flow of quickening, awakening and awareness. One invites the next and then yields to it. Focusing on awareness spirals one back to the beginning of another related level of knowledge.

A Little More Awareness of Awareness

Never underestimate the power
of compassionately recognizing what's going on.
— Pema Chödrön

In order to trust what body and self have to reveal to us, we also must trust that we are ready to be receptive. We need to believe we will not overstep our own boundaries of self-protection. We will not hurt ourselves, but rather experience meaningful healing from the release of cellular memories.

It has been my experience this is so. I have never regretted remembering aspects of myself through Yoga and Yoga Therapy. Some of the knowledge I have gained from my practice, from my body, has been joyous, some has been humorous, some has been painful, and some has been difficult to accept (such as shame and rage). But I have never hurt myself. I have never wished I could go back in time and not know. After the laughter, tears, discomfort or resistances, I have always been completely grateful for all of the quickenings, awakenings and awarenesses.

Self-knowledge does not push through the protective barriers of the ego. Instead, it waits patiently just on the other side of the door not yet cracked open. The authentic self is patient. There is for the self no time but the present. There is no limit to its ability to wait for ego to develop trust.

I have also observed in others – students of Yoga or not – similar self-knowledge availability. As someone once said, "When the student is ready, the teacher appears." I have also heard this said, yet I cannot remember who said it: "There is no way to push the river; equally you cannot hasten the harvest." I think we all have different points of readiness for different awarenesses, different thresholds of awareness.

In fact, modern science is beginning to hint that thresholds of awareness might exist physiologically (a concept my body already knows to be true). I first came across such research in an article from *The Journal of Somatic Experience* by Ian J. Grand, in which he discusses the idea of tissue thermostats. The article is written from the perspective that our body tissues take on the experiences of early life and shape us according to the character armor that results. According to Grand, the relationship between such tissue organization and the emotions these tissues contain controls the range of sensation and feelings we can access. Our tissue state allows us to experience certain things and not others.

Whatever has caused our tissue to organize on our behalf, our bodies form the context within which we then can or can't experience the world and ourselves. Grand writes, "Many feelings, behaviors and crises . . . can be seen as arising from difficulties in living the tissue state they have formed." We have, he suggests, organized our body "in order to not feel specific kinds of sensations in various parts of our bodies." We have set the thermostat of awareness at a certain level, which we are not willing to look beyond.

What Grand said next really caught my attention. He said, "There is a process of learning in which the tissue is addressed and taught in terms of its capacity to handle various kinds of movement, feelings and expressions." Although he does not offer what this process might entail, it is obvious to me (from my experience with my own body) this it at the heart of Yoga. The practice of Yoga is one that gradually and consistently re-sets the body's thermostats, shifting the thresholds of awareness potential. Over time, we come, said Chödrön, to "trust the living quality of energy" within and around us.

The concept of thermostats and thresholds is not a new one. As a personal fitness consultant I have long been aware of body thermostats and set-points related to weight loss and gain. In this case, the body desires easy maintenance, to remain a certain weight. There are also thresholds of aerobic capacity, the levels of work the body is currently capable of producing without undue fatigue. These are real limits, detectable through sensation, which can be changed by adding just the right amount of stress to the threshold. So it makes sense that our capacity for awareness might operate in a similar way.

I once attended a lecture by Daniel Goleman. He has performed vast amounts of research on the relationship of meditation, brain chemistry and brain function. During the lecture he referred to his concept of "emotional set-point" and of how our capacity for the happier emotions is enhanced by the practice of meditation. His theories of emotional set-point are based on the phenomenon called "neuroplasticity" – the way in which brain tissue is capable of continually transforming itself according to repetition of nervous tissue recruitment, such as the recruitment patterns that may occur in thought or in meditation. Much in the same way muscle tissue hypertrophies (grows in size and strength) according to the muscle fiber recruitment in exercise, brain tissue and, perhaps, the entirety of our nervous system, shifts our capacity for emotion.

All of the above, as well as my own experience of how I have become increasingly able to allow sensation and its meaning as it appears in my body, leads me to believe that we do have highly effective set-points for awareness. I also think these set-points are not permanent, and whatever their source in our physiology, they do not prevent the sensations of quickening. Curiosity, courage and choice can shift the thresholds of awareness. Yoga and Yoga Therapy are two very good ways to do this.

Silence, Presence, Breath and Spontaneity

Silence, present moment awareness, breath and spontaneity play important roles in the unveiling of self. They are all integral aspects of a Yoga practice. Each in its own way supported the emergence of my "loose ends" and my "secret breath" in the Yoga Therapy session mentioned above.

The self must know stillness before it can discover its true song.
— Robert Blum

The first time I really noticed the effects of silence was when I was hiking the Long Trail alone. Miles of walking, day after day, alone with my body . . . my thoughts and feelings; I moved in and out of long periods of silence. Sometimes the woods would be so quiet (especially if it was foggy), that I would feel as if I were silence within silence. I also remember moving in and out of many different feelings in that silence. Sometimes it felt completely natural and welcomed, and other times I would be gripped with unexplainable fear. Sometimes I was blissfully happy, and other times I sadly wept. There were moments when I felt a part of the community of the forest and others, when I felt achingly alone. In every scenario, silence had a lot to do with what I was experiencing.

The old adage, "Silence is golden," is true. In silence, it becomes possible to listen, watch and feel. In silence, the usual noise and chaos that we welcome as self-distractions melt away, leaving us to meet the truth of how we are the way we are. I have experienced silence as both peaceful and uncomfortable.

As if it were a magnifying glass, silence enlarges the sensations of being embodied so that focus and realization can more easily occur. Silence can accompany both movement and stillness. For me, however, the most powerful magnifier has been the partnership of silence and stillness.

Silence and stillness are cornerstone aspects of the practices of Yoga and Yoga Therapy. They support the creation of transformative space (internal and external) and accentuate the potential for self-discovery. Yet, for us in the West, silence and stillness have acquired meanings, which make these ways of being difficult to practice.

When I was growing up, I learned to associate silence with certain things that later stood in the way of an easy relationship with myself. In my family, silence was a way to show anger and contempt. My parents did not yell. If they were angry, they clammed up, which I always supposed was worse than yelling might have been. It seemed as though, with yelling at least, I would have a way to know what the anger was about. With silence, I had to hope I could figure out what I had done wrong. From this I learned silence was uncomfortable. It was something to tiptoe around while I waited for it to pass. I also got very good at the silent treatment of anger and hostility myself. I had good teachers and learned well.

Later, as I came to read and understand my body more completely, I realized that my ability to be in silence was distorted because of these earlier circumstances. I had to relearn the difference between silence and anger in order to feel comfortable. But more was happening at the same time. Silence had also become a way of avoidance.

As I got older, as I approached the mature body that I felt was the cause of so much pain, I found it helpful to become invisible. If I could just disappear maybe certain people would just forget about me. If I could just be quiet enough . . . silent enough, then I could be invisible. I remember hiding silently in my bedroom, listening down through the heating vent at the conversation in the kitchen, and huddling in my mother's bedroom closet. Just be quiet. Don't breathe too loudly – Secret Breath! Before that I even remember being four or five years old, sitting under the round oak kitchen table, holding the bells on the laces of my red shoes so that no one would know I was there.

Silence and stillness became my ways of disappearing. So as I entered Yoga practices, more and more I had to remember how to remain present in silence rather than invisible. I know this old need to disappear has a great deal to do with my current desire to write about being here, being embodied as a way of knowing one's true self.

Disappearing became my way of survival. I learned how to leave my body when being in it was too hard to bear. When the unwanted hands and tongues of others were on it, I simply could go somewhere else. Temporarily robbed of my body, I protected myself by not being present. This was, I think, a great act of courage and strength on my part, the best I could manage with the tools I had. I watched myself from a distance, separate from the pain. When I re-entered my body, I found it difficult to make sense of the way my body hurt because I had not been in it. It was as if I were coming home to a messy kitchen not knowing who had made the mess.

All of these experiences became part of my cells – my memory – and for many years I wondered about the constant low level of pain and uneasiness, the quickening. It was in silence and stillness that I was able to awaken and revisit the trauma of my past, and in doing so, was able to remove my desire to disappear. At first, my desire was to run from silence, from my body, from any anger still hiding there, my muscles tense and ready. Other times, I would float away, disappearing into avoidance of what was happening.

I kept wondering about compassion, openness and non-judgment – those qualities of transformative space. What did that mean to me? What did I need to do, or more importantly, what did I need to stop doing in order for me to move toward the sensations I was experiencing? Over time I discovered it was okay not to run. My unsafe body of the past became the safe ally for transformation. In coming back to my body, I began to more fully appreciate what could be learned by staying 'home'.

The physical postures of Yoga keep me in my body. Every day through my practice I reclaim the aspects of self that I imagined were stolen from me, when I was younger: worth and power. The less clouded wisdom of my authentic self tells me being here now, soaked in the brine of being human, is an experience not to be missed. This life, this richness of emotion and wonder, I think, is heaven, if there is one. The authentic self cannot be recognized until the grief and joy of being human are welcomed. One of my dearest teachers, Martin Prechtel, often says, "Your grief becomes your beauty." It appears I have come full circle back to this because, when I was young, I believed it to be the other way around.

After all this time, especially the time spent getting to know and make peace with silence, I think I may have finally stopped running. I feel a growing groundedness through my legs, a soft opening in my chest and a lightness in my stride. Movement is much easier. If I have not yet completely stopped, at least I can notice those moments when running seems like a good idea, and I can make a better choice. I like the way my body feels when I stop running and stay home. The physical ease of it is profoundly delicious.

The way to become comfortable with silence and stillness is to practice being silent and still, to enter into each with the intention of allowing cellular information to surface. While it is a simple concept to grasp, this is not so easy to do. In order to be still and silent, one has to let go of defenses and open to vulnerability. In order to know one's truth, in order to be visible, the layers of the ego have to soften into thin garments of light. In letting go, one comes to know and understand silence, which is a primary aspect of the authentic self.

Mearyn's Story

Even though I knew that Mearyn's life had been overcast with confusion and conflict, I could only imagine what was happening inside her six-year-old body that summer afternoon.

The elder of our middle daughter's children, Mearyn was visiting our front porch along with my other two granddaughters. Having witnessed her parent's hopeless attempts to remain a family, which included several traumatic episodes, she had begun a pattern of behavior that reflected her frustration with the way things were. Not particularly affectionate by nature with anyone other than her attentive Mom, Mearyn had grown more withdrawn and angry. This day, in particular, she was having a hard time being in the world of sharing and interaction.

There had been several fights over those small incidents that fill the world of tired children. Mearyn sat with her arms crossed over her chest, obviously beyond reproach. Another grandmother had kindly arrived with pizza, and cousins and aunts were bustling around setting up a feast on the picnic table. "C'mon Mearyn, have some pizza. It's your favorite! You'll feel better if you eat. Everyone else is going to. Let's go!" They cajoled her, patting her head and waving a slice in front of her angry face. I chose not to participate. Their methods felt out of place and poorly timed. If alone and angry was what she wanted, who was I to take her from it?"

It was clear to me that Mearyn had just plain had it. I could see the steam rising in her eyes. She was having nothing to do with the well-meaning prodding that must have felt like another assault. I allowed her to stay where she was and headed to the kitchen to distract myself.

The porch door slammed a moment later, and I saw the blur of Mearyn run through the house to the laundry room. I ventured after her and found her curled up on the floor, facing the corner between the dryer and the wall, wailing loudly. I crept up and squatted down behind her, expecting her to jump up and run away. Instead she curled up even tighter and continued to sob.

Silently, I placed my hand on the center of her little back and waited, no words – just my presence, hoping that my being there might somehow support her to be just as she needed to be. I saw no need to make her feel better, even though it was difficult to watch. My sense was that she needed to feel whatever it was that she was feeling – really feel it, and thereby justify her experience.

After a few minutes, she turned around, crawled into my lap, laced her arms around my neck, nestled her face into my shoulder and cried even louder. My body flooded with a grandmother's emotions and gratitude for being included in her world at that moment. In her six years this granddaughter had never before held me in this way. I was overwhelmed by her willingness to finally let me in.

Still . . . no words. I stood up and carried her to a chair. I was longing to offer ways of fixing . . . longing to soothe . . . but I offered only my silence, my still touch, my breath, myself. The others walked past now and then, trying to tease her into happiness again. "Not now," I said, and they left us alone.

After about ten minutes, Mearyn's sobs had shifted to the halted inhales that follow a child's big release. Then silence. Her breath relaxed. More silence. I sat very still, and so did she. Then, all of a sudden she sat up, all messy and red-cheeked, her face broadening into a huge light smile. I smiled back and smoothed her long brown hair from her face. She slid down from my lap, her release complete for now, her feelings validated, and ran off for her share of the pizza and the company of her cousins.

If I never again have the opportunity to use silence, stillness and presence, this moment, beyond all others, showed me the simple healing power inherent in these three ways of being.

Being Here Now

Awareness knows what's going on while it's going on.
— Stephen Levine

Everything occurs in the present, even remembering and looking ahead to the future. The present includes the new experiences of the moment as well as the re-examination of the past and future intentions.

If we are here now, we are in our bodies. The more distant we allow ourselves to get from what is occurring right now, the less embodied we become and the more anxiety we produce.

As you might imagine, being present was as difficult for me as was being silent and still. For the same reasons, remaining present took some intention and some practice. In my body I noticed how these three phenomena went hand in hand. If I were unable to be still, then presence was difficult to maintain as well. But I realized through my practice of these things that I could remain present to my unwillingness to be still and, in doing so, learn a bit more about what was behind the unwillingness.

What's Happening Now?

The simple but incredibly profound question that is the cornerstone of Phoenix Rising Yoga Therapy is "What's happening now?" This open-ended question is used in sessions to bring focus to anything and everything that is occurring in the present moment. It is offered from the intention of supporting the receiver to notice his or her experience while he or she remains present in his or her body.

Asking this basic question throughout your own Yoga practice (or throughout life's events) helps to keep you in your body and present to what you might discover there. In the asking lies the assumption that the answer is there somewhere in the mix of present moment experience.

Trusting that the answers are there is one thing. Having the courage to find out what they are is another. Time and time again, on my journey to discover myself, courage has been required. Perhaps this is so we eventually can come to know ourselves as the innately powerful beings that we are.

Being present may just be the ultimate courageous act. Everything, including quickening, awakening and awareness, happens in the now. Amrit Desai said, "Living in the moment, however, is the most dangerous situation anybody ever faces in life, because everything you have ever avoided is revealed to you when you live in the moment."

Breath

To treasure breath is like loving your face and your eyes.
It has never been unattainable.
                    — Master Great Nothing of Shug-Shan

Breath is more than the air as it is taken into our lungs and later exhaled. Breath means life, but not solely because we cannot exist in the embodied state without it. Breath also opens the doors of awareness that will lead us to life's richness.

At the onset of the Yoga Therapy session I have been describing, I was not at all aware of the "secret breath." By turning my attention to my breathing, I was able to discover something quite important related to my "loose-ends" state. I benefited from the simple observation of my breath. I did not try to change it, to breathe the way I thought I *should have* been breathing. I allowed it to be what it was and focused on it, as it was. I waited and allowed its message, "secret breath," to enter my awareness.

It is part of a traditional Yoga practice to become aware of how one's breath can be used in two ways. The first way is to observe how one's breath may be a reflection of one's current state of being. The second is to encourage what is universally known as a full Yogic breath, one which enhances the flow of *prana* or life force within the body.

From the root words "pra" which means first unit and "na" which means energy, prana is the limitless, formless, animating energy of the self and all things. Its purpose is to be known within and to move freely throughout bodies. As with cellular stories, prana can be felt in the body through silence, present moment awareness and, especially, through breath.

To feel prana in the body is to feel one's individual realness. Describing what prana feels like is as difficult as trying to describe the taste of honey. Words like "sweet" or "sticky" come close, but you just can't know the taste of honey without eating some. Prana is this way. We begin to recognize the way it feels through focused breathing just as we begin to recognize the taste of honey by taking it into our mouths.

Another way to feel prana is to imagine one of those days when everything goes right. No matter what, the events of the day flow into one another with perfect synchronicity. This is the way in which prana would prefer to flow through us, unimpeded and welcomed everywhere in the body. A body with fully flowing life energy feels, to the best of my descriptive ability, like an overall awakeness or aliveness, like a cellular wide, subtle, animated buzz.

There are also those days when one or two things just don't go smoothly, despite best efforts. Some processes get stuck, and things don't move or flow the way they could. Tensions and blockages in the body created by emotions and cellular memories can block the flow of prana and what is experienced is a sense of being bound up or closed off. Full Yogic breathing can begin to clear parts of the body that, for one reason or another, have been cut off from receiving the flow of life force.

A Yogic breath is a natural breath, even though breathing fully does not seem natural to most westerners. The natural breath is effortless, uninhibited, wavelike, rhythmic, calm and regular. It originates in the core of the body rather than high in the chest. Each exhale dissolving into silence, where the inhale breath will be spontaneously re-born.

The primary muscle of natural breathing is the very intriguing diaphragm. This large dome-shaped muscle separates our heart and lungs from our digestive organs. As it expands and draws downward, our lower ribs expand, inhaled air moves into the blood rich areas of our lower lungs, and our hearts and other internal organs get a bit of a massage. As it contracts and moves upward, air is effortlessly expelled in exhalation. The diaphragm will function involuntarily whether we focus on it or not and will also respond to our voluntary efforts to control or direct our breath.

In the absence of our intention and without our full awareness, diaphragms and breath become reflective of our emotional and stress states. Both have been described as gateways or bridges which allow us to become aware of and connect to our present moment feelings.

Sensations such as anger, fear, grief, sadness, impatience, anxiousness, boredom, happiness and relaxation can be brought into focus by observing the origin, quality, quantity, balance and ease of breath (as compared to the natural breath). Perhaps this is possible since sensation happens within the network of body cells, and "it is the cells that desire the breath."

Drawing awareness to breath, observing how it is occurring (or not) in the present moment within the space of silence and with the intention of spontaneous receivership, one opens the gate to experience and knowledge. Each exhale breath can then become a letting down of the drawbridge, connecting us closer and closer to the seemingly far banks of self.

Spontaneity

If we are ready to be with silence, willing to stay present and able to observe breath, the process of awareness begins to deepen. We are moving toward receiving, interpreting and integrating the messages of the body. We are lifting the layers and peeking at our authenticity.

A certain degree of spontaneity is required in order to become a better receiver of the material of awareness. Awareness is not a process that can be planned. Any assumptions that we try to make about ourselves, any expectations for outcome, only get in the way of true knowledge.

True knowledge evolves from a willingness to receive information in whatever way it wants to come – as a feeling, a sensation, a thought, an image, a memory, a color, a sound, a smell or a taste – followed by a letting go of censoring, editing or otherwise cleaning up what comes. The spontaneous allowing of information, no matter how confusing or scary or ridiculous it might seem, works to our advantage. Whenever awakening and awareness were welcomed in a spontaneous manner, clarity is always the next gift.

The Rest of the Story

Of course, there was more to the Yoga Therapy session whose thread runs through this chapter.

By bringing deeper focus to the *secret breath*, amplifying it, and bringing it more present, I was able to identify the place in my body where I was actually experiencing it, my solar plexus (just below my breast bone). The tightness in this spot (which I was calling, *Secret*) was shortening my breath, holding back every other one. Somewhere underneath Secret was an intensely warm, open area which felt like *Fire*. Fire was producing my fuller breaths that were mixed in with the secret ones.

I moved from a seated position to rest supine on my back. I realized that when I focused on Secret, my left arm felt constricted and drew inward toward my center. When I crossed my left arm over my chest, compressing the secret spot, I was able to discover that Secret was there to protect me from pain in my heart. Quick breath equaled restriction and protection. When the practitioner pulled this same arm out to the side of my body, the feeling of Fire became stronger. I recognized it as a profound strength that had been growing in me throughout my Phoenix Rising Training.

As I moved back and forth between the arm positions that amplified Secret and Fire, I came to this understanding: When Fire stayed strong, it could do the work that Secret had been doing for so long, but Fire could serve my heart in a confident self-secure manner instead of in a protective way. Secret had been trying to get my attention because she was afraid that I would forget to feed the fire of confidence once my training was complete.

I turned onto my belly, which compressed my solar plexus into the floor, making Secret even more pronounced. The sense of restriction here became very uncomfortable, the shorter secret breaths happening with more regularity. I could feel the suffocating nature of Secret despite her good intentions to protect my vulnerable heart.

My fellow practitioner then assisted me into a full cobra posture, which allowed Fire to blaze through my opened heart. I stayed here for several minutes, enjoying the sensations of strength and confidence as my body arose to meet the things that might hurt my heart. I realized those things were coming from me rather than at me – humiliation, disgust, abandonment and pain. As I recovered down from the cobra and sat my hips back to child pose, it became clear that letting go of these self-directed tortures was one of the things that would continue to feed Fire and keep her strong.

As I rested in child pose, both Secret and Fire could be equally present. Secret had a chance to be equal to Fire and was in this way honored for her important role as a protector of my heart. In Phoenix Rising posture, with arms reached up and out, the sensation of Fire moved into her fullness. As I returned to sitting and refocused on my breath, I found that Secret Breath had not disappeared, but it was happening only now and then. Much had been accomplished, and there was more to look forward to.

And Even a Little More

In the spring of 2001, about one year prior to receiving the above Yoga Therapy session, I had been in a head-on automobile accident. Today, when I see the photos of my demolished car, I have a hard time understanding how I came to walk away from it with minor injuries (whiplash, cuts and bruises). While I certainly felt the surface effects of this event in my body, I had no idea at the time how profoundly it had affected me in more subtle ways. It was not until the fall of 2002, several months after the session, that I was able to connect even deeper to my secret breath.

I was practicing my Yoga alone, watching my breath. It still had a secret. My shoulder, which had been severely bruised in the accident, had been bothering me all day. I even had gotten a massage in hopes of giving it some relief. As I continued to move through Yoga postures, I also noticed my hips were aching. This, too, felt familiar. Flashes of the car accident started to enter my awareness. I began to remember how I felt when I realized that the other car was in my lane. I remembered the sensation of the impact. I remembered the way I had braced myself, the helplessness, the fear of being hurt and the panic I felt as I dragged myself out of the car. I said out loud to myself, "I have been holding my breath since then . . . pushing my shoulder up since then . . . arching my hips since then. I'm still waiting for the impact. I can stop now." Secret Breath was gone.

CHAPTER 7
EDGES

*She tried the porridge in the big bowl and it burnt her tongue. Then
she tasted the porridge in the middle sized bowl and it wasn't
sweet enough. So she tried the porridge in the little bowl and it was
just right. So she ate it all up.*
— from *Goldilocks and the Three Bears*

In the practice of Yoga, as in all aspects of life, it is useful to
recognize and understand the concept of edges – the reality that there
is a place of 'just enough, not too much and not too little' in everything
we do. Edges describe the delicate thresholds of experience through
which we must pass at our own time, in our own way, so we may bring
our authentic selves fully into this human life. There are no limits to
the bounty of self-knowledge available at edges.

Perhaps edges are best described as a measure of allowing or
doing in relation to movement, sensation and virtually all experience.
If I am at my edge, I have the accompanying sense that to allow or to
do more would be too much. At the same time, I can see how allowing
or doing less might be unproductive.

Edges and Comfort

Just right edges are not necessarily comfortable nor are they
unbearably uncomfortable. They are places of sustainable sensation
where underlying meanings can be explored through focused
awareness. Edges are ripe with the potential for self-knowledge and
transformation. As with the just right porridge, an edge can taste like
the thing we need to nourish us in the present moment.

Formatting the words on the page in this "landscape" mode is a little edgy for me. I'm assuming it might also be a little bit edgy to turn this book and read it sideways. My intention is to be a little more at an edge while I am describing this concept and, at the same time give you a chance to share the sensations of this while taking in what I have to offer.

To experience another simple edge in my body, I place the palms of my hands together, interlacing my fingers. One of my thumbs ends on top of the other one with my fingers alternating each other down to my little fingers. This is likely how I always, automatically fold my hands. Without thinking about it first, the same thumb always comes out on top. If I part my hands just enough to unlace my fingers and reposition my hands so the other thumb is on top and all the other digits line up according to this new beginning, something interesting happens. I am instantly at an edge. The discomfort of experiencing this small act that is different from my usual pattern of doing things is surprising! My urge is to put my thumbs and fingers back the way they were, but I am able to keep them in the new position long enough to explore the accompanying sensations. I discover how little it takes to feel the effects of change in my body when I am paying attention.

Exercise

Place the palms of your hands together and interlace your fingers. Notice which thumb is on top. Now, spread your hands apart, just enough to unlace your fingers. Reposition your hands and fingers so that the other thumb is on top and all your other fingers line up accordingly. Observe how that feels. Do you have to fight the urge to put your thumbs and fingers back to the way they were at the beginning of the exercise? Pay attention to the accompanying sensations and feel how something that actually seems so insignificant can have such an impact on the rest of your body.

Learning About Edges

At first, my discoveries about edges were about pacing; I learned how not to over do or under do exercise and movement. As a personal trainer, it was my job to help my clients figure this out for themselves as well. When I was hiking the Long Trail, I certainly needed to observe my body for signs of overuse. But it was Yoga and Yoga Therapy that gave the concept of edges a whole new meaning.

This learning process began by simply feeling the edgy sensations of muscular fatigue as I entered and held Yoga postures. I noticed that sometimes I could find the place of balance, where I was neither holding back my potential strength nor was I pushing my body to extremes. I also began to notice my physical ease in postures when I could find this just right edge of effort. I was more likely to accomplish the postures when I recognized and was able to stay with these edges of sensation.

The more I played with the muscular edges, the more interesting they became. Certain postures seemed to bring up certain thoughts and feelings, depending on the edges I chose. It was as if muscular edges were the music to which my emotions could finally begin to dance. I needed to learn how to find the just right place of emotional sensation as well. How much emotion was I able to allow? How much personal information was I willing to reveal without overwhelming myself? Which places were I ready to visit? How long was I willing to stay? Which layers would come to the surface of my body . . . this moment . . . during this breath? How far would I open the door of my awareness today?

The following example from my journal is one of playing with a physical edge that taught me more about my relationship to conflict and struggle:

Another revelation in cobra: I got into it by keeping the posture very easy today – by not trying as hard. I discovered that the middle of my back, the stuck place, is related to the fear of my shortened breath in this up curve of cobra. I flashed on suffocation – on being held down with a hand over my mouth – can't breathe – I harden against IT – against the world, as it had been at that moment. I held my breath and hardened my heart. I thought, "If I can just get past this spot . . . rise above this point . . . then I can hold myself up and breathe!" At the low part of the posture there is no edge of breath. At the middle part of arising – huge edge! Then the upper part – full cobra – no more edge. I get stuck in the middle, and I continue to get stuck when I meet resistances/conflicts, suffocations of any kind. I can use my gift of self-compassion to move around those times when I am stuck. I can go easier on myself as I work through this.

Edges as Meditations in the Line of Love

I found being at an edge a bit like pondering the rim of the coin of duality. We are somewhere between right and wrong, good and bad, up and down and many more polarities. Edges present us with the opportunity to peek around the many sides of our experience. They are unique present moment meditations. Asking, "What's happening now?," while I am exploring an edge, causes answers to flow effortlessly into my awareness to the extent that I am willing to be receptive. Michael Lee writes about his experiences with edges in this way: "I was able to enter a state similar to what I had previously experienced in meditation. As I became the witness to myself, I was able to feel the uncomfortable yet inviting feeling of entering a void where images, sensations and even new awarenesses would come to me. I was not the doer of the posture; I was the receiver."

Stephen Cope tells us that edges contain the "potential to discover the real." Certainly, I *am* able to see more clearly through the layers of my ego by exploring my personal edges. As I deepen my exploration, my body's edge sensations expand and contract. Gradually I experience a fuller awareness of being alive.

My favorite description of being at an edge came from Pema Chödrön. She wrote that when we are at the appropriate edge of experience, it should "feel like a genuine act of kindness to ourselves." When the right edge is discovered – comfortable or otherwise – "compassion begins to spread by itself." We can choose to work compassionately with our edges, especially when they are a little shaky, chaotic or tender. In doing so, we are choosing the path toward transformation, Robert Frost's less traveled road. Edges must have the quality Goldilocks found in the bear's domain, so we can muster just enough bravery to test the porridge. When I work with my edges in this way, I realize I am practicing the art of self-love. In my practice and my day to day life, when edges present themselves, I move toward them, recalling these words from Martin Prechtel: "Never flinch in the line of love!" Hold the edge in favor of compassion.

A fellow Phoenix Rising Yoga Therapy practitioner recounts her story about sitting with an edge:

> *I was raised in a patriarchal family by an authoritarian and very critical father. During my childhood, to keep peace, I learned to please others at all costs. Thus I lost the ability to relate to my needs, suppressing my feelings and, instead, developed a pleasing, smiling personality.*
>
> *One day, in my Yoga practice, I mindfully entered a seated posture, began to notice intense sensations in my right hip and chose to stay with them. Although the sensations at times were almost unbearable, I continued to breathe into them. Suddenly, deep angry feelings raged throughout my body. My body shook uncontrollably*

as tears streamed down my face. I recognized all the years of stuffing down my feelings and literally "sitting" on them. I had tapped into an emotional complex consisting of self-rejection, self-denial and self-repression.

The Shifting Nature of Edges

Every new balance represents a capacity to listen to what before one could only hear irritably, and the capacity to hear irritably what before one could not hear at all.

— Robert Kegan

Exercise

Sitting tall, either in a chair or cross-legged on the floor or a cushion, keeping your hips facing forward, extend your right arm out in front of you at about shoulder height. Straighten your elbow and turn your palm downward. Rotate your body from your waist to your right, turning your extended arm as far behind you as you easily can. Moving your arm slowly, watch your hand as you move. Discover the amount of twist your body is ready for right now – your twist edge. Place an imaginary mark on the wall behind you to help you remember where your fingers have pointed in this first rotation. Then turn both your arm and your torso forward again. Now practice this rotational movement repetitively, disregarding the landmark on the wall and moving to what feels like your body's edge at each turn. Staying at each edge for only one or two seconds, make six such turns. On the last one, stop and hold the edge again, placing a new imaginary mark on the same wall. You may be able to see on the wall and feel in your body how your edge has shifted to a new spot. The quality and intensity of this last edge may be similar to those of the first one, but you have probably moved further than before. If you had tried to turn this far on your first attempt, the edge may have been too uncomfortable to maintain.

When you focus on the sensations of your edges, in whatever form they take, they shift in intensity. At first they seem wavelike as you zero in on just the right amount of sensation. If you focus on the sensations, they sometimes grow in intensity. As you pay attention, the edge expands and, with it, your awareness of its meaning. Then you need to make choices about the depth of sensation that keeps you at your edge rather than past it. Sometimes the edge moves too far, becomes too intense, and you may need to move back from it. Other times the edge softens, as in the rotational example above, and a new, deeper edge is attained. Softening is more likely to occur when you let go of arguing with the edge, or of trying to make it less, or of trying too hard to figure out its meaning. The messages behind edges are found as often in their softening as in their fullness. Each cycle of finding, focusing, deepening and softening can draw you closer to self-understanding.

Q.S., psychotherapist shares her following experience with shifting edges:

> *Six months have passed since Jim told me that he was HIV-positive. I am again at the Omega Institute for Holistic Studies, this time at the winter workshops on St. John in the Virgin Islands. I am here with my sister, Carolyn. I am here against doctor's orders. A week ago I pulled a muscle in my back. I was in bed for two days unable to move. My doctor advised me against this trip, fearing the inadequacy of St. John's medical care. Desperately needing relief from the stress of dealing with Jim, I insisted on going. I have arrived on St. John without further injury, with the help of porters and Carolyn. "I'll bet this is stress-related," I confide in her. "It feels like I'm carrying the weight of the world on my back."*

Carolyn is one of the only people with whom Jim has allowed me to share his diagnosis. In the mid-80's in Virginia AIDS is a dirty word. I suspect that this is based upon fear of the unknown. Jim is afraid that he will lose his clients, even his license to practice as a psychologist. This secrecy has become a burden for me. When he leaves work early feeling weak and light-headed, I must fabricate stories for clients and staff about migraines and flu. Our co-teaching used to be the delight of my work life. Now, however, the vicissitudes of Jim's health transform what used to be fun into playing a role. I look into his eyes, scanning for signs of exhaustion. I notice when the blood seems to drain from his cheeks. If I see his energy flagging, I step forward and take over the training. Surreptitiously monitoring him is mentally, emotionally and physically draining. Meanwhile, I pay little attention to my own needs. They have to be secondary to Jim's. "Jim isn't the only one who needs healing," I muse as I feel my strained back and my heightened anxiety level.

The more I talk, the more I walk, the more I do Yoga, the more I dance, the better my back feels. The doctor has cautioned me to lay still. Here I am wringing out my back with twists, extending it in forward bends and shifting the relationship of vertebrae with side stretches. After a week of Yoga every morning, I am pain-free. The movements are done so slowly that I can feel the tension in my shoulders, back and neck dissolving. Through this gentle stretching, I begin noticing the toll that my anxiety has taken on my body. I begin paying close attention to what's happening internally. Mid-week I am no longer thinking about Jim. Instead I am focusing on my body's positive response to the Yoga. This is what being in the moment is about.

I meet Denise Taylor, a movement therapist who uses improvisational theater, dance, meditation and movement to access what she calls "the authentic moment." With the afternoon sun streaming into our workshop space high above the trees and the sea, Denise slips The Blue Danube Waltz *into her tape deck. "Let your heart lead you," she encourages. "Set your heart free. Let your body follow as your heart's dance partner."*

At first my heart feels heavy. If I follow it, it leads me in a downward spiral toward the ground. I respect the urge, lying on my belly, covering my face with my hands so that no one can see my tears. I hate to cry. But no one seems to be looking. I roll into a ball, face-down, and sob. It feels like a volcano has erupted inside me. I taste wave after wave of salty lava on my lips. These waves seem to begin in my belly, wash through my heart and out my mouth and eyes until no more tears are left. When I finally stop crying, my body grows quiet. I feel drained, tired, like I could lie in this spot for eternity. I'm aware of how much I have held these feelings inside, and how they have kept my heart hostage. After several moments of still rest, my heart wants to dance. I stand up, feeling lighter, more open, freer and fluid. My heart leads me to leap across the floor as I did in ballet class as a child. I twirl with glee. It feels like that explosion of tears has unplugged some tightly held tension in my diaphragm and heart. I feel exquisite joy in this moment. I have not felt like this in months. I have forgotten what that feels like to unleash such rapture. I rejoice . . . at least for now.

Later in the week I again let my heart lead me into uncharted territory. This time it is during a Phoenix Rising Yoga Therapy workshop. Carolyn is physically supporting me in a heart-opening cobra posture. As I lie on my belly with my arms stretched behind me, wrists held by Carolyn, heart open, I fly into a rage. I growl like a tiger. Strange sounds seem to be traveling from my belly's deep recesses upward through my heart and out my mouth. I am not even aware of the source of my anger. I am just angry . . . furious. I have until now had an intellectual awareness of my anger – angry at God, angry at Jim. But I have only talked about it. Like the crying with Denise, this experience taps into a feeling – anger – which I haven't allowed myself to express. My body is wiser than my mind. When the fury subsides, I tuck into child's pose. I am lying in a small ball. My throat feels scratchy, my body limp. Carolyn's hand is on my back. Its warmth pierces through the space between my shoulder blades as if she were massaging my heart. Again, my body sheds wisdom about my life. This kind of support has been missing lately, and I desperately need it. Jim's secrecy around his illness has isolated me. I leave St John committed to asking Jim to let me share his health problems with a wider circle of friends. I decide to ask for more hugs. I am dedicated to paying closer attention to my body's messages.

Stephen Levine writes, "When we have compassion and patience enough for ourselves to let a state come up and be seen, it slowly disintegrates." My experience has been that my edges do not shift when I impose assumptions on their meanings. This also happens when I avoid the truth about what my body is trying to tell me. I remain stuck at my edges until I get out of my own way. If I can let go of my assumptions and avoidance tactics and simply and spontaneously allow myself to receive the edge's meaning, it will change and take me to the next level of self-inquiry. "Only when we accept what is happening – no matter what it is – can we choose where to go next or how to be with it. "Playing the edge," says Michael Lee, "involves exploring the fine-tuning that takes us even deeper into the experience, be it a posture or in life."

Edges Everywhere

Edges that arise during the postures and meditations of a Yoga practice or a Yoga Therapy session have a way of shifting into daily life. As I practice finding my edges on my Yoga mat, I get better at moving this skill into the walking, talking, being, doing aspects of every day. The more i learn about edges and how to be with them in a useful way, the more I can notice them everywhere, as with the following example of simply sitting in a cafeteria.

I discovered another new edge today, a really big one! I was looking for a place in the cafeteria to sit for lunch. I sat down between two friends and started to eat. My seat was in the far end of the room, so most of the other customers were behind me. I was sitting so that I was facing the back wall of the room. There was no one sitting across from me – just the wall. From where I sat, I couldn't see what or who was behind me. I became so uncomfortable! I felt my heart harden like it did in practice this morning. My throat tightened. My breath shortened. I wasn't enjoying the conversation around me. I began to sweat more. This felt like fear. I was feeling vulnerable, in need of protection; I needed to be able to face what might be coming. I couldn't deal with it. I was too tired to sit with this edge. I got up and moved to sit with my back to the wall. I think I'll try again tomorrow and see what happens then.

Michael Lee writes, "Once an awareness comes through the body it has already started to happen in life. It is not just a thought. It is an experience of a different way of being and so the learning is almost automatic. Those changes have been much easier to take fully into life than anything I may have read or heard or thought about." I have found this to be true through my own body in my own life. I no longer separate my on-the-mat practices of Yoga and Yoga Therapy from the rest of my life. It is all one thing – the way I discover myself to be while I'm on the mat is how I can potentially be everywhere. Lee adds, "Without an edge there is no growth, no learning, and no change. Too far back from the edge is boredom and atrophy. Too far out from the edge lies self-destruction. The edge, in both body and life, is always moving. It is always expanding outward into unknown areas."

Edges Avoided

Had I known then what I know now about edges, I wonder if my Long Trail Journey might have ended differently. As I go back and read my journal entries from the last few days of the hike, I can feel again the longing and the pain in my body. I was at some pretty big edges of awareness, and I was full of resistance toward them.

About sixty-two miles shy of the Canadian border goal I had the adrenaline packed experience of being chased several yards by a full grown mother moose, who decided quite assuredly I did not belong in any proximity to her calf. I ran downhill to avoid her wrath with my fully loaded backpack (about 50 pounds worth) thumping against me. Later, having successfully escaped, I scared myself with the thought of how injured I might have become, and how I might have been stranded for a time before any other people came to my aid.

Later that same day I hiked over mountains that demanded much of me. Several times I had to lower or hoist my pack with ropes so I could negotiate steep slabs of rock. There were also ladder climbs, steep drop-offs and ravines that challenged me to the point of tears. At the end of the thirteen mile day was a long, toe-bruising downhill that seemed to never end. When it did, I told David (who had hiked in from the North to join me for a few miles) I no longer wanted to be alone. I asked him to come with me from there to Canada. He agreed.

Although I appreciated his company at the time and always will love the wilderness experiences that we shared, I realize now this invitation was my way of avoiding the edges that were being presented to me. I often wonder if I asked him because the edges were really too big, or if I asked him because the edges were just right, and I did not yet know how to be with them. Still, I have to acknowledge everything about this experience unfolded perfectly. It eventually led me to explore more about the edges that began to emerge that day.

The following is from my Long Trail journal on the final day of the hike. When I read it now, I feel again how I sensed I was somehow cheating myself out of the experience edges, and how I blamed myself for not being good enough to face them.

"I could have gone on by myself. I could have been fine by myself. I'm angry because I didn't give myself that gift. I said I wanted to do this alone and I didn't make it all the way. Even though I did most of it alone, I broke my process with the whole thing and now what do I do to get that back? How do I replace

this pain with joy? Maybe not replace it but evolve it. I imagine how it would have been if David or I had suggested that he leave the trail at the last highway crossing. If we both had joyously understood that the last stretch of this journey was mine – and mine alone – to finish. If I had taken that last walk in quiet, writing . . . feeling . . . crying openly instead of holding back, how would my completion of this trip have been different? If David had said, 'Go ahead. I'll be waiting for you at the end', and he had been there like that, with his wonderful David happy tears in his eyes to see me make it, how would things have been changed?

I felt nothing when I crossed that border – my thunder stolen – my fire defused – by myself! How could I do this to me? My pattern once, though, would have been to use my fear or pain as a reason to completely stop – to give up. At least this time I did not give up. I did walk the whole way. At least I discovered that pain can be a reason to continue. I will need to find a way to end this journey with the sense of self I went looking for.

To take off my pack causes me pain because the journey is not ended – or do I want it to end. I am different, but how so?"

CHAPTER 8
QUESTIONING AND LISTENING

The spider brings the web out of herself and then lives in it.
— Ramakrishna

If you bring forth what is within you, what is within you will save you.
—Jesus, *The Gnostic Gospel*

The experience of quickening calls for attention. Once I decided to turn my awareness toward the sensations, emotions and thoughts of quickening, it became clear I would need to make certain choices. Was I willing to allow my awareness to deepen? I was ready to ask, "What's happening now?," but was I ready to listen to the flow of answers from my body? Did I want to know the truths about myself? The choice was completely mine, and for the first time I realized no one else was going to judge me accordingly. It would be alright either way.

I was drawn to my choice to listen because I knew I would not hurt myself by doing so. I might, however, hurt myself by turning away from the potential within self-awareness. The road ahead was not clear nor was it smooth and fast-going, but it did feel safe. The choice to move forward required my willingness to meet the parts of myself that, for once helpful reasons, kept standing in my way. The process was simple. All I needed to do was say "yes" instead of "no." As Eva Pierrakos wrote, "It means ingathering yourself; calmly, quietly wanting to know the truth of this particular circumstance and its causes. Then you need to quietly wait for an answer."

All Yoga begins with witnessing, evolves through questioning and listening, and matures through receptivity, understanding and integration. Sensation, thought and emotion are watched, accepted, unfolded, acknowledged, and brought honestly into the light of daily life circumstances. Then the cycle begins again with new quickenings and new levels of awareness. All is a process of divine timing, each morsel of self-revelation offered and received in relation to readiness.

Respectful Inquiry

If you want to become eloquent, don't begin by talking. Listen.
— Martin Prechtel

Asking a felt sense is like asking another person.
You ask the question and then you wait.
— Eugene Gendlin

In my twenty years of work as a personal fitness and health consultant, it is my observation that Western culture individuals have some difficulty with genuine self-respect. Our tendency, myself included, has been to live out a sort of embodied battle between the high, self-imposed, cultural expectations of perfection and the aches and pains of suppressed, understandable human suffering. The body is more frequently considered as a thing that needs to be continually fixed according to current standards. Listening tends to turn into avoidance, diagnosis and medication. To this we add the fact there doesn't seem to be enough time in the day to pay attention to the sensations of quickening, much less actually explore and expand awareness of self.

I have discovered respect to be, perhaps, the most valuable aspect of successful self-revelation – respect for body, respect for self, and respect for all the ego parts that allow us to negotiate the world. I think that in order to be able to learn about oneself, in order to lift the veil from the authentic self, respectful inquiry is needed. And the origins of such inquiry lead to gradual understanding and clarity – "the unfolding totality of being."

I have come to imagine self (both my authentic divine essence and my individual human 'parts') and body as sages or elders who deserve the same, if not greater, respect as any other great teachers. So how does one treat such sages? Again, in the West, this seems to be a forgotten custom. Elders are often pushed aside rather than given a place at the head of the table.

When I was growing up, I often heard the words, "Respect your elders." But very few of my adult relatives earned my respect or my trust. When I began to question my body, I found I really didn't know very much about sincere respect. Oddly, it was by admitting to my lack of knowledge about respect that self-respect began. As I continued to observe this old disservice to myself, it gradually became clear that respect was made of right intention, clear listening, patience, receptivity and gratitude.

Eloquent Asking . . . .

*Ask yourself how your life is going and quite soon
you will have a bodily felt sense.*

— Eugene Gendlin

. . . . Of Sensation

One way a quickening or any other sensation in the body can be asked is, "Who are you? What is your purpose? What teaching do you bring?" Phoenix Rising Yoga Therapy practitioner L.M. asked her body in the following way:

During my first experience with scanning my body for information about myself, I became very aware of a pain in the right side of my back near my shoulder blade. It felt just like a knife had stabbed me there, but I questioned why it would feel that way and who would want to do that to me. At first I could think of no one. And then I realized that my ex-husband had stabbed me in the back by having an affair and leaving our marriage after 13 years and 2 kids. I cried, sobbed and soon calmed down, realizing the pain was gone.

. . . . Of Emotion or Thought

The same questions asked of sensations can be asked of an emotion or a prominent thought or belief. In this case it may be helpful to add the question, "Where are you in my body?" or "What sensations are present along with this emotion, thought or circumstance?" Such is Soleil's story:

> I have chronic pain in my shoulders. It has been getting consistently worse over the past five years – ever since my divorce became final. I have worked with this struggle with allopathic doctors, physical and massage therapists and chiropractors during all this time. In the past few months I have started questioning the metaphysical aspects of having shoulder issues. Articles that I've read talk of things like "carrying the weight of the world" on my shoulders, but this isn't something that seemed to connect with me.
>
> And then, this past week I decided to get a cranial-sacral massage. The therapist put me in a very meditative state and started the work. He lifted my arm gently – so slightly that I almost didn't even know he was moving me. And when the shadow of my arm crossed over my eyes, I tightened up – just waiting for the pain that I knew was going to occur. Only what came to me was a word – PROTECTION. Ahh . . . what was that again? Protection. That was it!
>
> I left the table and spent the day wandering about considering that word. What did I have to protect myself from? When was I not protected? And so I began the process of moving backward in time. What has come to me since then is the realization that I have never been protected. My father was not available for me in this role, and my two older brothers were off doing their own thing when what I really wanted was for them to notice me – and protect me. I remember one evening when I was 16. My oldest brother played in a band and, lucky for me, I looked old enough to get into the bar. I got picked up by this guy at the bar. I remember that I wanted my brother to intervene – to come to my rescue and

tell me not to go home. But as I left the bar on the arm of this drunk man, all I got from my brother was a raised eyebrow and a wave of the hand. I was so sad. I did go home with this guy, told him I was underage, and left as quickly as I had come.

I have gotten used to taking care of myself, but it has been weighing on my shoulders, and, ever since my divorce, I have to protect my son, too. And now the real work begins. I have the awareness. Body shifts are slowly beginning to occur. Now I thank the aches as they become the physical reminders of my internal healing process.

. . . . Of Circumstance

Asking can also bring focus to a life situation, issue or problem with the simply profound question, "What's happening now?" Watching the body for related felt sensations may lead to understanding or even to solutions as it did in Rose's case.

I have had a long and interesting relationship with my mother. I am 55 years old now, and she is 82. She was not at all a typical 1950's mother. She went back to school, got her degree, and began teaching biology at the same college she had attended. She has always been a strong role model for me, and I am grateful to have grown up with the belief that I could do anything I set my mind and heart to. I was fortunate to live near my parents when my own children were young. Well, fortunate and challenged. In being witness to my mother's relationship with my daughters, as well as with me, many of the edges and rough spots in our relationship were brought to light.

It all seemed to come to a head about fifteen years ago. I realize, in retrospect, that my mother was coping with a very difficult transition from her many years in a rich teaching career to retirement. I think transitions are difficult times for most of us humans – they are a place of the unknown, the unfamiliar and change (a very tough thing for someone who likes to be IN CONTROL). Yes, that's my mom – in capitals! During this time 15 years ago, I was experiencing such difficulty in being in relationship with my beloved mother that I actually thought we needed family therapy. I couldn't imagine doing anything without her participation. Fortunately for me, I learned this wasn't true, and my practice of Yoga and learning from my body came to the rescue!

By lucky chance, I was scheduled to attend an advanced Yoga teacher training during the thick of this hard time. It was two weeks long. I decided to also schedule two Phoenix Rising Yoga Therapy appointments during the training. Smart move! During the teacher training, I became aware of an area in my body – in my right hip – that was holding so much tension. I had a feeling it was somehow connected with what was going on with my mother, but didn't really know what all that meant. And, I knew that my Phoenix Rising appointments were going to offer me an opportunity to explore this in depth. The day of one appointment, I had reached such a physical and emotional peak from all the Yoga we were doing in our training. Well, I knew just where things were happening in my body, I knew how to access that physically, and my emotions were so present. I began to order my practitioner around – "do this, do that!" (Who likes to be in control you might ask?) My practitioner wonderfully supported me in all of this through touch, posture choice and simple dialogue. What I encountered in my right hip felt like a big snarly mass. The image that came to me as I stayed with the sensations and all they evoked was a house. My mother had set up house in my right hip. "How dare she! Breathe, breathe." What followed was more staying with what was happening and more release of tears, anger and holding.

The clarity that emerged was that I was the one who had erected this house. My mother didn't live there, but a part of me that was so like my mother did. And that was the part of me that was feeling so triggered. Recognizing this gave me a brilliant opportunity for choice. Did I still need all that – my own need to *control? How did it serve me in the past and was it still serving me now?*

My experience is that our bodies provide such clear and honest access to our Selves. In this situation, being supported in deep physical and emotional opening provided an opportunity for real change. The upshot is that my relationship with my mother changed profoundly. I don't know that her behavior changed, but my reaction to it changed completely. Because my reactions changed, so did she. It was like learning a new dance. I like this one much better.

. . . . Of Self

When the answers seem to be coming too loudly from ego parts, another way of asking is to invite the authentic, always wise, ever present self for insight and advice. The embodied, authentic self can be asked for its whole-being universal observations, which is what I had done in the story below:

I had been feeling really angry and victimized that circumstances were preventing me from my daily routine. I had not been able to practice my own Yoga asanas or meditation. I was called to be on task at home, work, and study – no end or break in sight. I was stuck inside with the weather. I felt deprived, discouraged, and pissed off at everybody and everything that I thought was standing in my way. Sitting still one morning, these words of wisdom became clear: "My life was my Yoga practice!" (Duh!) All these edges were my Yoga postures! I was being given the opportunity to practice every minute rather than an hour or two a day! How could I possibly be angry at such a gift of time? And in fighting it, I had been wasting it! Suddenly, everything started to make sense. It was like some dam broke and the water of consciousness poured over me.

So now, as each situation arises, I am able to remember, 'Okay. I'm practicing my Yoga. What's happening now? What or who is this edge? Where am I willing to work within this edge?

Tell me more about all that. What stands out as being important here? How does this show up in my overall life – or not? What do I take from this? How will I integrate this experience into my life? What can I affirm? What needs practice? What does the part of me who knows without thinking have to say about this? When is it time to come away from this edge for now? How will I accomplish this?'

Had I not arrived at this simple realization, I believe that I might have remained stuck in a discouraging victim's perspective.

Developing Eloquence

Whether we are asking a felt sense, a feeling, a circumstance or self, it has been my experience that the process of self-awareness deepens according to *how* we ask. When we ask from a place of clearly wanting to know, without the limits of expectation, then we will find out. On the other hand, when our agenda is to hear what we want to hear instead of the truth, then the truth will remain veiled.

If we ask begrudgingly, sarcastically or demandingly, our bodies are apt not to respond. If we push, insist or try to beat our bodies into submission with the intention of getting rid of symptoms or discomforts, then sensation, emotion and knowledge remain locked inside our cells. When we behave this way, we add even more pain to our tissues.

In my Yoga practice I prefer to move slowly and deliberately from posture to posture. I have learned the benefits of inviting my body to move, *asking* muscles to engage *versus* telling them to. I invite the edges of sensation to become more present as I explore strength, balance and flexibility. When I force my body, I struggle, and I blow past any possibility of self-discovery. When I slow down and respectfully ask my body, there appears to be no limit to what it will tell me.

I also discovered I needed to come to my body bearing self-created gifts. Gradually I set aside masks, pretensions and expectations, showing up more naked, holding fewer weapons, until I could come with the most humble offerings: respect and willingness. In the beginning, it seemed more questions than answers arose in my body. When I began to ask more simply and eloquently with less of an agenda, the answers began to flow.

One day last spring, I was walking in the woods near my house and found that an old logging road was flooded by the run-off of melting snow. Since I had never seen this happen before, I decided to have a closer look. The spring stream, which normally crossed the road and ran naturally downhill toward the swamp, had been re-routed by someone. Stones had been set to divert the flow of water down the road instead. This did not seem right to me. It was obvious the stream wanted to go its normally unobstructed way. It seemed sad and confused, and watching it made me feel the same way. I felt a little catch in my throat and in the front of my hips. It felt like stifled expression and halted progress.

I walked down to where the water would normally go and found a diverse pattern of three-wheeler tracks tearing up the dry ground. Since it was my property, and I was more interested in nature's fulfillment than the speed satisfaction of adolescents, I went back to the little dam and began to remove the rocks. Immediately the stream began to flow the way it was intended to. It was joyous to watch! The water sung louder as each stone, stick and clump of leaves was tossed aside. The catch in my throat dissolved, and I began to sing with the stream. When I finished and stood up to watch the excited water making its way to the swamp, I noticed that my hips were also fine again.

I thought, "This is how it is with the flow of life in me. This is how it is with the flow of information through my body." As with the water, my path flowed clear as I removed the disrespectful stones, which I unknowingly had placed in my way.

Intention

> *It is part of the cure to wish to be cured.*
> — Latin Philosopher, Seneca

An important aspect of respectful inquiry is intention. Intention is not goal-setting; it is more open ended. It is a reflection of readiness. It is stating with clarity the degree of one's willingness to receive in relation to the questions being asked. For example, one might state one's intention this way: "I am ready to look more deeply at the message of the pain in my right hip. I would like to receive any information that might help me to understand how this pain is serving me, so I might eventually let it go. It is my intention to learn something from my hip."

Earlier I wrote about the old adage, "Be careful what you wish for." My intention to hike the Long Trail certainly led me into more than I had bargained for at the time. The power of intention is great. As soon as we put forth what it is we will allow to happen, it begins. Yet, unlike goal-setting in which we have a picture of a more precise outcome, intention often sets us out on the unknown road. We have asked a clear question, we are ready to learn the answer, but we do not know what it will be.

The following demonstrates how the power of intention led Laurie to begin to address long-held body tension regarding life situations:

During a recent Phoenix Rising Yoga Therapy session I found myself in an Assisted Knee down Twist posture. The practitioner asked, "What's happening now?" I talked about how I was feeling an incredible sense of perfect balance and complete relaxation. It was so blissful that I never wanted it to end. I had never experienced anything like this before. I had an image of a teeter-totter and I was right in the middle, with arms outstretched, in complete balance. My intention for this session was to explore the difference between control, surrender and giving up. Even though I know intellectually that surrender does not mean giving up, a part of me feels like surrender is giving up. At one end of the teeter-totter was control (right side) and at the other end was giving up (left side). Here I was right in the middle. What was this place? It came to me that this must be surrender. It was a feeling of not having to do anything.

The practitioner then asked me to say more about giving up. I thought "if I give up then I might as well be dead." As this thought settled I had a sick feeling in the pit of my stomach, and I

started to feel a shift in the balance of the teeter-totter toward the
left (giving up). I started to panic, not wanting to lose this perfect
place. I was so afraid of losing this feeling! I tried to take control
and hold on desperately to this place of perfect balance. The teeter-
totter then shifted over toward the right. Tension started building
up in the muscles of my body especially in my right leg (this leg
was injured a couple of years ago and continues to be a source of
pain for me). As the tension increased in my body so did the pain
in my right leg. I then started to let go of the control and the teeter-
totter started to go back to the left and the tension and pain began
to ease up. I'm trying to find that middle place, but I can't seem
to find it! As the teeter-totter starts to shift even more to the left,
I again try and take control. The tension and pain increase. As I
teeter back and forth the tension and pain become very intense. I'm
now holding on so tightly that the tension and pain are continuous.
I have reached my edge, and I no longer can stay in the posture.

What did I learn from this session, and how does it show
up in my daily life? Over the last couple of years I've had some
stressful events and changes in my life. I've been trying to stay
in control to protect myself from emotional and physical pain.
At times I've been so tired and angry I've felt almost like giving
up. If I give up, I might as well be dead. This intense desire
to control and protect myself creates a great deal of muscular
tension in my body. I am at a point where I'm unable to let go of
this tension. It is chronic, and my leg pain is chronic. It appears
that all I need to do is surrender. It seems so simple, so why is it
so hard?

Wanting Results

Orientation toward results can distract from the "in the moment process" of authentic awareness. If we have a particular result in mind when we set our intention, then we will see what we want to see, hear what we want to hear and most likely not get the point that our bodies are making. Instead, we need to let go of outcome and welcome whatever is there.

For example, if my aim is to get rid of the pain in my hip, I am saying that I am not willing to receive the message of the pain. Demands have been made, but no respectful questions have been asked, and no answers are likely to come. I sometimes wonder if this is one factor that leads to chronic pain. Does the constant resistance to self-knowledge in combination with results-oriented wishes increase the volume and frequency of trapped discomfort? On the other hand, if the pain does go away through such an intention, it will likely resurface with greater acuity or in a new location. I have said, "I wish this pain in my hip would just go away." My body has responded lovingly and accommodatingly. "Okay. Here is a different one in your foot. Is that better?"

"There is a paradox that if you aim at the gains you are likely to miss them and if you forget the gains then they are at your feet," says Shankar. The problem is we want the gains. We expect the gains. We feel entitled to the gains. We want to make them happen as quickly as possible. In a culture where instant coffee takes too long to make and computer printers are too slow, the idea of letting go of outcome is not easy to do. Yet, I have discovered that I gain more when I do let go. The self-truth that comes from open-ended intention is always far richer and more beneficial than any goal oriented results that I might have imagined.

It remains important to seek traditional allopathic medical care for pain. My suggestions for asking and listening to the body are not meant to replace needed health care modalities. Instead, I offer that we can consult ourselves while we consult others. The combination of inner and outer asking, followed by listening, is a powerful combination. The trick is to find health care providers who will listen *with* us and not only *to* us.

Listening With

I listen to the wind, to the wind of my soul.
— Cat Stevens (lyrics from *The Wind*)

One of my mentors in the Phoenix Rising Yoga Therapy realm, Achalan Gene Barnett, shared with me his wisdom of "listening with." This concept shed a brighter light on the process of respectful inquiry.

In relationships there is a subtle yet important difference between "listening to" and "listening with" another person. If I listen *to* you, I separate myself into the role of consultant. My tendency might be to offer advice or to try to fix something. I hear you speak, I make assumptions based on my own experience, and I may even think you are expecting me to come up with the answer to your plight.

However, if I listen *with* you, if I simply hear your words along with you while you are speaking, I validate your experience by bearing witness to it. My silence helps enhance the transformative space you are creating and honors your process as it presently is. As you speak out loud, and I listen with you in a non-interfering way, then you may be better able to hear yourself – your own body and wisdom – and so come upon your own answers.

Upon learning the concept of "listening with," I discovered I could apply the process to my own Yoga practice. My practice deepened as I became the silent witness to my own process, as I listened *with* myself.

"Listening with" is the essence of what Yoga calls "witness consciousness." It is the way of being that leads us into the state of "jivan-mukti" or "soul awake in this lifetime." The witness, who listens with the individual human aspects of myself, is my authentic self. She sanctions all of my human conditions and experiences from a non-dualistic, non-judgmental, compassionate stance. From every cell of my body, she remains still in the eye of the hurricane, which is my life. My witness self watches my humanity with uncensored, impartial endurance. She "watches, but does not . . . participate," knowing "All this is me . . . an activity of my being," and at the same time remains joyous in the knowledge that she is also divinely, universally free from the human process.

The witness, who listens *with*, accepts both her divinity and her humanness. She is the heart of my being, my embodied authentic self. She cultivates the two primary aspects of witness consciousness: "clear seeing" (the intention to pay attention) and "equanimity" (the knowledge that everything is already okay).

This is Bob's account of how "listening with" led to self-awareness:

> *I had been experiencing a dull, throbbing ache in my upper buttocks and hip area. In a long-held, seated, forward-bending posture, the stretching out of my upper buttocks was absolutely wonderful. It allowed me to observe the variety of sensations that were underneath the dull throbbing. These underlying sensations were lively, interesting, noisy and sparkling – anything but dull! I didn't want to come out of the posture for quite a while because it felt so good to be free of the throbbing and to have this variety of sensations instead. As I stayed in the pose, I got the connection between this experience and the probability that my depressed personality masks a sparkling and lively inner self.*

Permission Not to Know

> *Actively feeling means turning our attention minutely*
> *toward our moment-by-moment experience,*
> *dropping what we think about what is happening,*
> *our evaluations and judgments about it,*
> *and becoming fully absorbed at the level of sensation,*
> *feelings, and energy.*
>
> — Stephen Cope

> *In the beginner here are many possibilities,*
> *but in the expert there are few.*
>
> — Zen Master Suzuki Roshi

In order to learn anything it is helpful to be comfortable with not knowing. If we already know, then what is left to learn? Respectful inquiry is not possible if we already think we know it all. It is even more difficult if we think we are supposed to know it all. Yet, in admitting we don't know, we show our vulnerability. We might make mistakes. We might not be perfect after all. We might even be a bit foolish.

But what if we let ourselves off the hook of having to know everything? What if we give ourselves permission not to know? In giving myself such permission, I realized this was not vulnerability, it was freedom! I came to let go of my fear of foolishness and welcome the bliss of being the beginner.

Each Yoga practice becomes like the first when we come to the mat with the attitude of a beginner. Because we don't have to know, struggle is replaced by fresh opportunities to understand ourselves in the world. Expectations give way to exploration. Assumptions dissolve into realities. Judgments turn to self-acknowledgments.

The paradox is that through not knowing, we discover that we already know. By letting go of needing to know – by getting out of our own way – knowledge arrives. Getting out of our own way and not having to know is not playing dumb. It's not escaping or exiting or hiding. It's not an aspect of failure, giving up or giving in. It is about cleaning out a space in which learning and transformation can occur. The wisdom of the self exists in the "cleaned out space."

Patience

> *Do you have the patience to wait*
> *Till your mud settles and the water is clear?*
> *Can you remain unmoving*
> *Till the right action arises by itself?*
> — Lao Tzu from *Tao-Te-Ching*

Another important aspect of respectful inquiry is patience. While moments of insight sometimes seem to occur with lightning speed, we forget all of the smaller, more subtle awarenesses that prepare us to receive the bigger message. Wisdom is not a fast thing. Just as an old woman may happily stir a pot of slow cooking soup all day, wisdom likes to take its time. We are simmered, like the soup, over the fire of life energy, receiving continuous small dashes of seasoning (little insights).

Cultivating patience has something to do with relinquishing control. It appears as if it is human nature to pull and push, to struggle to make things happen when we want them to, and to prevent things we want to avoid from happening at all. With the practice of patience we learn to let things evolve at their own speed and in their own time.

Sri Aurobindo wrote, "In all Yoga the first requisites are faith and patience." Contemplation is at the core of Yoga, and patience supports contemplation. It does not work to be in a hurry. Even though we grow older, the essence of who we are does not recognize time in human terms. Body, having no agenda other than to support our human experience regardless of its length, watches no clock. Both exist in the present.

And being in the here and *now*, in the present moment, is not the same as what I call "the mother's now," as in "hurry-up and get to it because I say so" (a sometimes seemingly necessary discipline technique). We can not hurry the transformative process. Even when change seems to drop quickly into our lap, we can look back and marvel — sometimes chuckle — at the turtle-like slowness of the long line of learning events that preceded it.

Turning our attention toward body and becoming aware of how we are at any given moment is the best way to become present. With practice this can be done almost instantaneously. Yet the translation of present sensation usually takes more time. To hurry the process is to miss the truth. We are on the clock of divine timing after all. "To every thing there is a season."

Gratitude

The remaining element of respectful inquiry (although there are probably more I do not yet know) is gratitude. As I cultivated the previously mentioned elements, my gratitude toward the whole phenomenon of being both human and divine expanded. As I worked with each aspect of inquiry, respect and gratitude began to feel similar to the sensations of everyday miracles — they were part of something that was naturally 'right'.

On and off my Yoga mat, even during those times when I feel afraid, sad or lonely, I remain grateful. I'm grateful for the poetry of my body, the eloquence in asking and receiving, the power of intention, the grace of witness consciousness, the freedom of not knowing and the timelessness of patience.

An entry of gratitude from my journal, April 2002:

> *In morning practice I discovered a place of deep gratitude and sadness at finding the joy of self-essence in the space between the two spirals of my body – gratitude that I found it for a few seconds, and sadness at its illusiveness – for the moments when I forget it is there. But I am beginning to come to know each practice as a 'do over' . . . a chance to look again, to begin again, to remember what my humanness and the world around me calls me to forget – the possibility, the promise, the absolute, the ever present, ever constant grace – the always available self. There is never a point at which the do-over opportunities come to an end. There is always another one. I alone keep myself from remembering this. Only my fear will keep me from taking the next do-over. I'm the only one who ever thinks I don't deserve another chance at peace.*

The Poetry of the Body

The meanings that are acquired through direct experience are much more powerful than meanings acquired through conceptual thought.
— Eugene Gendlin

The body speaks in poetry. To a poet this is a simple language. To the analytical thinker, the body's poems may not initially be so easy to decipher, let alone assimilate into daily life experience. Over time, however, we can all become poets. It is possible to learn the sometimes quite literal and other times metaphorical language of the body and the self.

Once, I tried to put together the pieces of a puzzle without the benefit of the cover of the puzzle box. I had no way of knowing what the puzzle picture was going to be. It was difficult to bring the image into focus, to figure out how the pieces went together, but it was also possible. After a bit of discouragement on my part, I discovered it was more interesting to watch the moment to moment unfolding of the unknown picture than it would have been to match it to a predetermined box-top expectation.

Coming to the body as a poet or sage storyteller of self is somewhat like putting a puzzle together in this way. Difficult as it may be, setting aside expectations and assumptions clears the way for actuality. The images, sensations, colors, smells, tastes, sounds, temperatures, qualities, quantities, emotions, thoughts and energies we notice have meaning for our hearts only. There is no other puzzle in the world exactly like the one we are. The information stored in our cells and tissues is different from, though often similar to, those of anyone else.

One Phoenix Rising Yoga Therapy practitioner tells of a client who cast a first glance at her body's poetic puzzle:

N.B. is President of a New York City advertising agency. At age 53, she is intelligent, well-educated and open to trying Phoenix Rising Yoga Therapy. During a session posture, I asked "What's happening now?" She replied, "What do you mean?" I asked what sensations she was experiencing. She said, "I don't know." I invited her to tell me more about not knowing. She told me she was not aware of feeling anything from the neck down because when she was a child she had been confined to her bed for years and lived only in her head – reading, writing and imagining. Later, she never played or developed any physical practices. L.G. started to cry and told me she had been in therapy for twenty years and had never cried in any of her psychotherapy sessions. Connecting to her body again, she was able to begin to release long held emotions around her long illness.

As we begin to recognize the subtle and often metaphorical meanings in the poetic language of our bodies, transformation is already beginning. Even if we are resistant to what we are discovering, we can take slow steps toward change. Our experience of transformation will continue. The rate of change depends on where we choose to stand in relation to the experience of changing.

Poetry from my body in Knee-Down-Twist

In knee-down-twist, there is one side and then the other side of me.
The dualities of my physical body show me how to be (or how I am) with
the dualities of life and other people and of nature . . . of all.
One arm, the left one, feels like it is braided.
I feel the desire to comb it loose . . . let it move . . . offer it some fun.
Right arm always gets to do the fun stuff.
Maybe my left arm is not the only part of me that could use some fun.
How can I comb some looseness into my life? Hmmmm.

Synchronicity

Poetry and synchronicity seem to go hand in hand. I have observed how the flow of life circumstances and events, even the smallest of details, always highlight my body's messages.

Synchronicity, a term coined by Carl Jung, refers to those unifying moments when previously unrelated circumstances and people come perfectly together and re-orient an individual in some way. Synchronistic moments are felt in the body as energetic realities. There is often an eerie rightness to such events that seem to tie the loose ends of other confusing moments together, leading to clarity or perhaps new questions. When we are awake and aware of each incident, each moment of life, we see how they synchronize with our sensations, feelings and thoughts to perfectly form the lesson we are ready to receive.

A Learning Curve

It is helpful to know that even though the language of the body may be initially foreign to us, eloquence and comprehension improve with practice. The learning curve of self-understanding is not as steep as I thought.

According to Yoga philosophy we each bear the seed (*bja*) of contemplation. The seed already contains individual and universal potential for understanding. From quickening onward, attention, respectful inquiry and consistent listening, with or without enlightenment, prepare the seed of contemplation for germination. The more we listen, the wiser the body becomes.

W.M. shares his experience with the learning curve of understanding self:

My expertise as a child growing into a man was to close off my body and numb it so I would not be able to experience all the pain AND the bliss that was lurking just around the corner. This would manifest in my body by a collapsing of my chest accompanied by very little lung capacity. As a musician, I would have moments of feeling intense opening in my chest and my solar plexus while playing and chanting. During the times I was numbing my body, it was quite a challenge to fuel the unconscious desire to open my chest, express vocally through my throat, and have the courage to perform through my solar plexus.

The more I allowed myself to be in my body and experience all emotions, sensations and thoughts both good and bad, the more I was able to be more creative, connect more with other people, and truly feel the connectedness and oneness that I had read so much about.

My thoughts about not being worthy, or not being good enough, or hiding from my own light all came through my body, through poor posture, sunken chest and tension in my jaw and head. Through ten years of Yoga, I have been able to slowly and with time, patience, and commitment, unravel the physical patterns that have blocked me from living my full potential. For that I am grateful.

The more respectful inquiry becomes, the more the poetry of your body is allowed to flow, and the more you are awake to the synchronicity of life events and sensations, the more you will discover about the truth of yourself in this world. As Jack Kornfield writes, "Gaining enlightenment is an accident. Spiritual practice simply makes us accident prone."

CHAPTER 9
WORKING THROUGH
THE STUFF OF AWARENESS

The darkness is behind you; the daylight has come.
However, as always, you are put on notice to be mindful not to collapse
yourself into a future or to behave recklessly in your new situation.
A lot of hard work can be involved in a time of transformation.
Undertake to do it joyfully.

— Ralph Blum

The information that comes into awareness through our deeper observations and investigations of sensation, thought and emotion is bound to be met with some resistance. As I continued to examine the things I had been carrying around in my backpack, I encountered certain aspects of myself I did not want to acknowledge. But as I became aware of these unwanted qualities, I was also becoming increasingly aware of my inherent wisdom. When I turned as much to what I knew as to what I thought, I was able to learn how to self-mentor and self-sooth my way toward acknowledging the stuff of awareness. I could integrate, rather than cast aside, those qualities that once caused me to struggle.

Meeting Resistance

When we struggle against our energy we reject the source of wisdom.
— Trungpa Rinpoche

The first problem I encountered with the stuff of awareness was how to admit that I was resisting. At first, I was not able to see it was happening. I was unable to allow that I was creating a struggle, that I was controlling awareness, limiting myself on the spectrum of awareness potential.

I discovered that these things were happening during Yoga postures. I noticed my body struggling to be stronger or longer. I noticed struggle itself. I also began to realize that when I stopped struggling and allowed my body to find just the right edge – not too hard, not too easy – then I could more easily accomplish the posture. If I didn't control or avoid my body, I could easily find the just right positioning. I began to wonder how this might also be true in all other aspects of my life. What else was I controlling or avoiding? Would the postures of life become easier if I could let go of resistance across the board?

I found the process of removing resistance began as soon as I acknowledged its existence. Struggle softened in the light of awareness, and I began to meet the things I once believed belonged to others, but not to me, such as shame, rage, guilt and victimization.

I was able to say, "Yes, these things are present" but in a very detached way. I treated these qualities as unwanted guests. They were there, but I didn't have to spend time with them. They could just eat and go home. I could stop controlling their existence, and I could also continue to avoid them. I began to fall asleep, zone-out or disappear in postures. Even in the ones that required more muscular effort or balance, I would come to the end of the posture and not remember anything about it. In this way I came to know avoidance as something different from resistance.

As with resistance, as soon as I recognized avoidance, the process of acknowledgement began. I began the process of what Dan Goleman appropriately describes as the "spell of chronic rumination." "Okay, these guests *were* at the party. I was going to have to include them somehow. But how?" I chewed on this at length, at times slipping back into resistance and avoidance. "How might this be done?" Each day, each practice, I shifted throughout the spectrum of awareness in order to gradually find my way. In postures – in my body – I re-experienced struggle and disappearance, but I now could understand the reasons for both. I allowed emotions to flow without needing to fully explain them. I experienced some uncomfortable digestive problems. I began to realize that all were related to this rumination. What was the next step?

As I continued to move in the direction of removing resistances, my ability to listen to self-wisdom was continuing to grow. I was cultivating those seeds of consciousness as I was pulling out the weeds of history. I began to accept ownership of my less preferred qualities, to own my complexities. Begrudgingly at first, but gradually less so, I approached my more shadowy guests.

The poet Rumi wrote, in his famous poem *The Guest House*, "Even if they're a crowd of sorrows, who violently sweep your house empty of its furniture, still, treat each guest honorably. He may be clearing you out for some new delight." The poem also contains the line, "The dark thought, the shame, the malice, meet them at the door laughing, and invite them in."

Joanne offers her story of meeting and acknowledging intimate resistances through her body:

> *My body has for a long time been most reliable teacher. This has been especially true in the sexual arena. I have learned more about myself by noticing the conditions that support my body to open to receiving than I have in any therapy office or personal growth workshop (and I've been in plenty of both)!*
>
> *I am, by habit, a giver and a striver. Until I was 30, sex for me was about giving pleasure to my partner and receiving some vicarious enjoyment in the process. My own body was responsive only to a point. I found myself striving to have an orgasm, to give this to my partner – an effort that repeatedly didn't work.*
>
> *Years ago, with a casual lover, I found myself very responsive and easily orgasmic. I was amazed! Without particular effort, my*

body was taking me to places I had thought were inaccessible. At this point, I began to trust that my body did know how to open.

A few years later, in the context of a loving and committed relationship, I had the opportunity to experience my body functioning at various and very different points along the continuum of openness and receiving. The openings were sweet and sometimes ecstatic; bumping into the closed doors was usually excruciating.

I learned a great deal by watching the openings and the closed places and all of the surrounding terrain. In a nutshell, I learned that whenever I externally and internally access and act from a place of self-honoring, my body enjoys and easily opens to the loving ministrations of my partner. I discovered that the most common way I did not honor myself externally (with others) was to shrink back from speaking my feelings or needs.

As I have peeled back the layers of not honoring myself internally, I have discovered that underlying my striving and my doubts is a sense of unworthiness to receive pleasure, especially if someone is specifically focused on giving it to me.

Ironically, I find myself opening with increasing ease, frequency and enjoyment. My body has given me the clues over the years, directing me as I notice "warmer" and "colder." By listening to, and following these cues, I have chosen more self-honoring ways of behaving in relation to others. With people I love and trust, I speak more freely about what I want and how I feel. My body has taught me what it really means to love myself in very tangible ways. As I treat myself with more honor and respect, I am becoming a kinder and more compassionate human being.

Slow Process

It is always a danger
To aspirants
On the
Path

When they begin
To believe and
Act

As if the ten thousand idiots
Who so long ruled
And lived
Inside

Have all packed their bags
And skipped town
Or
Died.

— Hafiz

Though the process of greeting guests is slow, tedious, and ongoing, it is centering and calming to invite each one in for tea. To finally sit down with each one and get to know it, to get to know ourselves, is grounding. Eventually we can see the value of each guest, as well as how to host each one appropriately. Banishment does not work. Inclusion does. Over time, each satisfied guest shows up less and less. When they do show up, we can simply say, "Ah, here is shame. It is good to see your face again. I thought you had forgotten me. I know you well enough to also know you are here for a reason. Thank you for coming. How long will you stay? And, by the way, have you met my other guests, confidence and calm? You have a lot in common. Come. Sit here as long as you wish."

While it is helpful to welcome all of one's guests, it is also important not to become subservient to any of them. We need to be observant enough to know when one is taking over. We need to learn something about the dharma of each guest, their purpose in our life. Discovering this made it easier to have them around, and it also led me to realize it was no longer necessary to send out invitations. On one occasion, however, one particular guest passed away. The following experience occurred while I was receiving a deep tissue massage and dialoguing with my body.

Obituary, March 2004

Shame died peacefully in her home last night at 7:00 P.M. following a long struggle with illness. She was surrounded by her loved ones.

Shame was a local resident who played a significant role in the body-mind-spirit community where she resided for 51 years. She consistently played a part in, or was at the root of, virtually every community event and experience that occurred in her lifetime. She will be remembered as a strong catalyst for change; her contributions were not without controversy, which eventually led her community to clarity through the gift of confusion.

At the time of her death, she transferred her power to Self-Confidence, per her last will. Self-Confidence is quoted here: "I believe I have the years of experience and the ability to hold the responsibility that shame has carried, but in a new and different way." End quote.

As a testament to her years of contribution, shame left many journals and log books that are said to contain the history of her life and community roles. They also contain the story of her feminine lineage and her relationships to her children and grandchildren. These journals are already a greatly appreciated reference as new community experiences unfold.

Shame is survived by her family: Confidence, Dignity, compassion, Ego and Self and many other old friends and recent acquaintances.

A private service was held at the time of her passing. She will not be forgotten. In lieu of flowers, please dance.

Through the language of our bodies, our awareness of our personal stories and our inherent wisdom can continue to expand. Although the nature of resistance and the nature of our guests remains the same, what changes is reactivity. The more we say "yes" to guests and to the experiences of life, the more we can say "yes" to ourselves. The discomfort we feel along the way is not due to the process of change; it is due to resistance to the process.

Shadows

Jungian analyst Robert Johnson describes the shadow as the part or parts of us "we fail to see or know." Through the processes of suppression and repression, emotion, sensations, thoughts and actions take a back seat to circumstance. I consider shadows to be like children who have been stuck in such a back seat for a long ride. They are so ready to jump out of the car at the next opportune moment. They may sit quietly back there most of the time, but when they get the chance, they come through loud and clear. With the energy of penned-up children, my shadow emotions surprise and sometimes disturb me.

When uncharacteristic words fly out of our mouths or we are somehow stunned by our own behavior, our shadows are showing up. At those times when we look at what's happening and say "Who was that?" in regards to ourselves, it can be helpful to attempt to answer that question.

As it is with children, so it is with shadows. Living with shadows and understanding them requires endless patience. Yet getting to know one's shadows leads us in the direction of transformation. Although they may not be what we want to look upon and acknowledge, doing so usually "permits us to find gold in the dark side."

In order to fully understand self, shadows have to be seen, heard and felt. They are all on the guest list and must also be welcomed to the party. It is important to "relate to the shadow as a mystery, rather than as a problem to be solved or an illness to be cured."

When I was learning the techniques of Phoenix Rising Yoga Therapy, I received an unannounced visit from a strong shadow while working with a practice client:

As I witnessed my client's process in receiving this Yoga Therapy session, I could feel a growing activation. It felt as if my body were about to boil. I could feel the little bubbles forming near the bottom of the pot (my body). What I was noticing was very strong. I remember not giving it free rein. As a practitioner I knew this was neither the time nor place for this shadow to be revealed.

My client was talking about voices from her past – voices that said "You can't. . . . You look. . . . You act. . . ." Her voices were coming from the kids at school, who had taunted her as a child. My shadow was ready to jump out of my throat and land on the mat beside this client. This shadow was the biggest, strongest kid on the playground. Had there been one around, she would have grabbed a baseball bat and said "Okay, let's go get those assholes!" With or without the client's help, shadow would have held up each one of those kids by the collar and slugged them all the way to the outfield with one swift blow! "Take that and don't ever come back! Get out of my way. Get out of my body!" And the best part would have been watching those last few remaining kids run off in terror of that horribly swift bat and the strong-armed follow through behind it. Then my shadow would have turned into the wolf and howled at the moon. Then into a hawk in order to soar above those running kids, making sure they were gone. Next, my shadow would have turned into a breath and jumped back down my throat, and I would have come back full of adrenalin and gone to sleep, recuperating and basking in my glory.

Of course, none of this happened in the session, but I acknowledged I could only hide my shadow for so long. There was a bit of nobility in what my shadow wanted to do. Yet the childhood dragons I was imagining slaying during this carnage were my own. The cellular experiences I had, or wanted to have, in this session were mine and mine alone.

During this experience, my throat began to tickle, and I coughed uncontrollably for a few minutes. My eyes watered, and my breath was tight. This was all at about the time when my shadow of rage wanted to jump out of my throat. When the session was finished and my client had gone, my nose bled profusely, as if I might have been hit back by one of those playground thugs.

I went back to the mat. Here I am writing about this shadow. It seems enough for now to be acknowledging her presence. But I think tonight I will howl at the moon and watch what happens. If I do, I'm less apt to go looking for a bat.

My shadow is a friend and ally who is asking to be incorporated into my being. She has been hanging around for a long time, waiting for me to open the door. Now that the door is open, I see she is just like that little kid who the other kids told "You can't . . . You look. . . . You act. . . ." She is the part of me that wanted to defend me from the intruders of my past, but could not, at the time, do so.

I can see how I could use a little of this shadow's strong, clear, no bullshit attitude. I would like to be as present as that from time to time. I appreciate her honesty and her nobility. The ugliness of her rage is beautiful. It is my intention to discover ways of letting this shadow out, so she no longer has to lurk around in the background of my being.

Shadows of Light

Indeed it is the most difficult thing in the entire human experience –
to claim your Self, your Life, your Light, your Truth. . . .
— Emmanuel

There was, as I said, nobility in this particular personal shadow, which brings up the point that shadows are not always dark. We resist our nobilities as well as our dark sides. It is often harder to acknowledge the presence of wisdom consciousness, of inherent divinity, than it is to acknowledge the more rough human edges.

Shadows as Projections

> *This is a central fact of the human existential dilemma.*
> *In order to see ourselves, we must rely on reflection.*
>
> — Stephen Cope

> *You will recognize the outer 'enemy' as but a reflection*
> *of what you have not, until now,*
> *been able or willing to recognize as coming from within.*
>
> — Ralph Blum

Left unrecognized, shadows are usually projected onto other people through relationships. Projecting is the act of seeing within another person a thing that belongs to us. Whatever this thing is, we also see it as being directed at us from this other person, rather than as a reflection of what is actually in us. For example, you may get irritated by your boss's inability to properly recognize you for a job well done. You feel cheated and angry at being treated this way. You see the situation as something your boss is doing or not doing to you. But if you look closer, if you notice how this feels in your body, you may find there is a familiarity to what is happening. You may find you treat yourself in this same way. You may also see yourself do the same thing to others. Why should others get your recognition if you can't even give it to yourself? You are irritated not by your boss but by your own inabilities. You have seen yourself in your boss. He has unknowingly been your mirror. Your boss's behavior aside, you have projected onto him an image of your own and then blamed him for what you have seen to make it easier on yourself. Projecting is easier than owning.

"What we see in the other is, in fact, in us, or we would not see it." For me, coming to terms with projections has been the edgiest part of self-revelation. It has also been the most valuable. In recognizing the edges of self-responsibility for projections, I have begun to let go of blaming another for my feelings. In practicing this, we can begin to let go of self-blame.

Carl Jung suggested "we can be grateful for our enemies for their darkness allows us to escape our own." Throughout my journey along the trail of self-revelation, I bump into appropriate projection screens. Whenever I am in the process of questioning and listening to myself, I seem to run into just the right person who will help me to see more clearly. Synchronicity again plays a role in discovery. If I am awake, if I turn to my body and say, "What's happening now?" I will inevitably learn a great deal from each encounter.

Environments of Awakeness

There also exists a sort of reverse projection process. Not only can we see ourselves reflected in another person, we can see other people reflected in ourselves. In other words, if we arrive in an environment of awakeness – in the presence of another who is self-aware – we can recognize our own potential for self-awareness. The calmly abiding center of one self can evoke "the calmly abiding center that already exists in each of us in potential form." Knowing that abiding awakeness has blossomed in another adds compost to the quickening seed of consciousness in ourselves.

Providing an environment of awakeness is at the heart of Phoenix Rising Yoga Therapy. One essential component of a Phoenix Rising Yoga Therapy session is "loving presence." Similar to Carl Roger's concept of "unconditional positive regard," loving presence refers to the practitioner's supportive, caring and unobtrusive way of creating transformative space. Nothing is interjected to direct the client's experience or to remove them from it. The wisdom of the client's body is trusted explicitly; there is no outcome oriented plan.

The environment of a Phoenix Rising Yoga Therapy session models for the client a way in which they can support themselves. By being with, listening with, the client begins to learn how to be with, listen with his or herself. The "loving presence" aspect of Phoenix Rising Yoga Therapy has been researched and its importance documented by C.L. Kokinakis in *Teaching Professional Standards: Training Yoga Therapists in Loving Presence*.

Letting Go and Usefulness

At any point along the path of discovery it is easy to return to chronic rumination. When you notice this happening again in your body – in you –that there is something you are still hanging on to that is getting in your way. You may not be aware of just what it is, but you can usually find out by watching your body and your breath. When you discover what it is, it generally turns out to be something that has great value, but maybe not for the particular forward movement that you were intending to make. Within this sort of discovery there is often an element of humor. It's funny . . . the things we forget we are hanging on to.

I tend to have the habit of carrying too many bags to my car at one time when I'm traveling for work. I could make more than one trip, but I get lazy. So I approach my car's door handle with no extra hand to open it. One morning, as I was struggling to open the door without setting any of the bags down, my back and shoulder began to spasm. I froze for a second, thinking I may have injured myself, and in that same moment saw the metaphorical comedy being played out. Why didn't I just let go of something? Did I need to be holding all of this? I had with me everything I needed to get through the day, but did I need it all for the action of opening my car door?

The hilarity of this simple situation started me laughing. I sat down on the ground and had a good time chortling at myself. Then I realized the deeper meaning of this. There were likely other times in my life when I unintentionally sabotaged myself, my path, by traveling a bit heavy rather than light. After all, just because I might need a canoe to get across a river on my way to hike a mountain, this doesn't mean I also have to carry the canoe up the mountain with me.

We can choose to set things down. We can choose to see the humor when we forget to do so.

Crashing

There is no greater agony that bearing an untold story inside you.
— Maya Angelou

The path of self-transformation is full of natural emergencies. In the process of awakening, resistance and discovery, there were times when we just don't want to or can't know any more. There are times when we need to hang out with recent discoveries for awhile before moving on. In order to own and know awarenesses, we have to be with them. When awarenessess begin to pile up, we begin to suffer from chronic awareness syndrome.

While these times feel dark and heavy, they are not completely so. When I was in them – when they were in me – I could turn in the direction of my inherent wisdom for self-mentoring. Ram Das said, "Never are we nearer the light than when the darkness is deepest." The key is not to avoid the darkness, but rather to experience it, recover from the experience, let go of the need to self-perpetuate the darkness, and move on to new discoveries.

Self-awareness cannot occur without crashing. It is a normal part of the process. We can learn to come back to body and breath and use the question "What's happening?" or sometimes "What's not happening?" We can coax our bodies to tell us more, especially when we don't want to know. As we ask and answer, if we listen for the wisdom that is within this darker experience, it is always there. We can find the meaning in the crashing. Light and dark begin to touch each other. Light illuminates shadows, and shadows shift to make room for light. As we cultivate patience, we may find that what lies ahead is worth the present discomforts. The key is in finding the meaning. "One can endure any suffering if it has meaning; but meaninglessness is unbearable."

For me, one such crash occurred in March 2003:

> *I am resisting, suffering, integrating, and desperately seeking ground. I am riding huge waves of confusion and clarity, and there appears to be no loving presence to hold the space for me to do this work other than the space that I create for myself. It seems as though some unseen energy is holding me present to the difficult edges that I am experiencing non-stop. The intensity of these edges is so great – the crests of these waves are so high – that*

I am saved only by my breath and my faith that they are somehow necessary. Still, I sometimes want to be like Harry Potter and don my invisibility cape forever.

The more I try to ground myself, the more events and circumstances test my ground. My old ways and patterns of struggle, my old image of being the eternal victim, my old strategies of throwing the first punch – or at least hitting back – no longer work. Having invited these old aspects of being in for tea, they have softened, and their slow withdrawal leaves me feeling vulnerable. Allowing my vulnerability to join the tea party is strange – an odd mix of fear and peace. Surrender to vulnerability further confronts me with the never-ending task of being while doing, which brings me to even more edges, from which I re-visit the remnants of old beliefs, defenses, judgments and assumptions.

Everything from relationships to the frigid weather seems to be holding me in place – inside (both figuratively and literally). Every experience is inviting me to face every fear, anxiety and shadow. Every button I have is being pushed and every trigger pulled to a level of pain and grief that have, on many occasions, seemed unbearable. But they were not so. None of the mirrors that have been held to my face have broken. The things that are breaking are my resistance, my fight, my 'front', my excuses, my denial, my lies, my status as a victim and my feelings of responsibility for the way others are.

Each wave of pain is often followed by a wave of bliss – happiness so intense it strangely (and thankfully) balances the pain. This wave experience is similar to the moments after giving birth when all direct memory of pain dissolves away in the watery eyes of the infant you hold.

My sense is that the universe is providing me with a supreme opportunity to test my unfolding questions and beliefs. It is holding me present to this chosen path closely and intensely so I might actually get somewhere

My body is an important part of this process. Sharp, unusual pains in my joints and deep throbbing aches in my muscles and bones accompany this time of living between. They arise for no apparent 'physical' reason; there is no injury – no explanation for their existence except to demand attention to the reality that I am, in fact, in pain and to the ways in which I might choose to work with it. To ignore my body is to ignore the pain. Indeed, when I acknowledge the pain, allow it to remain until its message has been made clear, and address it, it goes away on its own. Clearly, the task is not to remove the pain, but to allow the pain to remove itself.

Depending on the quality and quantity of crashes, it is helpful to sometimes seek out an "environment of awakeness." To surround yourself with others who understand the process of self-discovery can enhance your ability to mentor and sooth yourself. To temporarily alter one's environment, without the intention of running away, can provide a different perspective on the uncomfortable processes of growth and change. Self-mentors often need mentors in order to remember, "I am okay. It's only change."

CHAPTER 10

INTEGRATION

Whatever our initial vision of spiritual life, to be authentic,
it must be fulfilled here and now, in the place where we live.
— Jack Kornfield

As we work through the self-information that arises in our bodies, a natural process of integration begins. Awarenesses interconnect, drawing together a fuller, clearer picture of the lesson at hand. Loose ends of experience move toward each other, completing the picture at least for the moment.

I once heard someone define nirvana, a Buddhist and Yogic term for enlightenment, as the state of being that occurs at the moment of seeing a thing through to its completion. Perhaps this is true. As the lessons of discovery merged into the foreground of my awareness and I accepted and found the value in new knowledge, I certainly experienced follow-up sensations of calmness and connectedness.

The process of integration is two-fold. First comes the somewhat untidy process of gathering all the sparks of awareness and the stumbling attempts to change certain aspects of self in day to day life. What eventually follows is an effortless, natural integration that gradually occurs through the synchronicity of those initial sparks. What at first may seem like loose ends become integral fibers in the fabric of change.

Natural Integration

Natural integrations are "ah-ha" moments. They are the dawning insights that occur because we have slowly added up the different aspects of growing awareness. However, as with other aspects of transformation, natural integrations need invitations. They follow intention, readiness and non-resistance. I realized my willingness (or unwillingness) to arrive at the answers was a guiding factor in the process of such insight.

As I began to realize the broader context of my day-to-day life as a never-ending, metaphorical Yoga posture, I also began to watch my body for information more consistently. The avenues of observation I discovered on the Yoga mat became even more valuable outside of my structured process. I could ask, "What's happening now?" at any time, observe my body, and discover something of value related to the life situation at hand. The techniques of awareness were clearly assisting me to be more fully present to life, helping me to navigate my own private wilderness.

Some Funny Things Happened On The Way Out Of The Forest

At this point on my journey three new awarenesses emerged. The first was that even though my perspective of the wilderness had changed, even though *I* was changing, the wilderness was not! I harbored some sort of hope and belief that those around me would easily understand what I now knew. Why wouldn't they? It was so clear to me. I also expected to find the loving arms of compassion all around me as I moved through the more difficult materials of my awareness. This was not usually the case. I discovered the aloneness of change and this, in itself, presented an edge.

The second awareness to emerge was my realization there was no end to the cycle of questions and answers. As if I existed under a never waning full moon, once I awakened to the process of discovery through my ever-present body, I could not fall asleep again. I tried! I remember writing to my mentor Karen Hasskarl, "I don't want any more FGO's (Fucking Growth Opportunities), thank you very much!"

Then I saw the hilarity of the situation and realized I could rest without being asleep.

The third awareness was the edgiest of all. I ran smack dab into the pendulum effect. I found out pendulums *do* swing both ways. Of course, I knew this from high school physics, but I had never applied the concept so fully to my life process. My swings in the direction of joyous fulfillment and self-revelation were balanced by equal swings in the opposite direction. The bigger my upswing was, the bigger my swoop down into new murkiness – my crash. At first, I imagined something to be wrong with my process. But after experiencing a few full swings, I remembered how one side is supported rather than challenged by the other. Both ends of the swing have an up curve. After spending some time at the town park actually swinging on the swing set, my body found the peaceful spot at the bottom of the curve. As with the coin, both sides of the "swing" were really one thing, and it was process.

The Wilderness and Me

It is sitting loose to life,
accepting it as it comes [that is the] pearl of great price
worth any sacrifice to attain.
— Geraldine Coster

Freedom means moving comfortably in harness.
— Robert Frost

For me the early stages of integration were a sometimes difficult process. Even though I realized the layers of projections I was making onto those around me, I still encountered a felt sense of disconnection in my relationships, in my joints. I found it difficult to describe my process to others. To answer the simple social inquiry "How are you?" seemed a useless endeavor. Within the walls of my own home, at work and in the company of friends I often felt as though I were someplace else. I had not disappeared; I remained present. But I didn't quite know how to speak, how to act, how to *be* the self I was unveiling. Even though I had taken off many masks, I was still at a masquerade ball.

At first I found it difficult to integrate the "slow way of initiation" — the process of self-transformation — into my current life relationships and obligations. My new perceptions of myself and others made it hard to remain comfortable with the status quo of my previously established place in the world. I found myself in what psychologist Keith Thompson refers to as the "ambiguous not-quite-here and not-quite-there . . . place of enormous fertility and spacious potential." Riding the spiraling wave of growth, I was sometimes living in the way things used to be and sometimes in the way things were beginning to be. The journal entry at the end of the previous chapter is one example of riding such a wave.

As I played with this new edge of awareness, what started out as difficulty became less so. It became enticingly interesting to observe myself both on the Yoga mat and off. I found that living between the old and the new presented me with the opportunity to step back, invite a wider perspective, and muster the courage to let go of assumptions. I was at yet another "threshold of adventure.."

Robert Kegan writes, "Experiences which challenge old meaning systems nourish development." I found this to be true. I remembered about patience and once again gave myself permission not to know. I remembered I was not the only one wearing masks. Through my observation of the ways in which I was embodying this process, I was able to become increasingly aware of the assumptions and conclusions I tended to draw from others. Gradually, I was able to begin to let them go. The experience of this sort of integration became grounding and settling instead of confusing and disconcerting.

I continue to invite integration to happen. The process involves taking on the dual tasks of continuing self-exploration and change in the midst of meeting the demand of life on a day to day, moment to moment basis. As new experiences continue to land in my body, as I continue to unlock the doors to my personal story, and as I steadily unveil my inherent wisdom, I am more and more certain of this:

"The final freedom is not freedom from the world. It's freedom in the world."

A Box-in-a-Box Gift

I found the ongoing, never ending process of self-revelation to be similar to one of those gifts that consist of a box within a box within a box. I remember receiving one of these for Christmas one year. I chose the biggest, most obvious box from under the tree and began to unwrap it. As I got excited about getting it open, I found another smaller wrapped box inside. Opening the second box, I found a third, and so on. I think there were five altogether. When I finally got to the box that contained the gift, I was delighted, but I was also left with the questioning feeling, "Is there more?"

The path I am following mirrors this experience. There is always another box. Each "next one" finds me more objective than I was before. I have begun to use experiences rather than to allow experiences to use me. As Joseph Vrinte writes, "Growth [is] a never-ending series of free-choice situations." Whether or not I open each box is ultimately up to me.

Swingin'

You cannot stay on the summit forever.
You have to come down again. . . .
One climbs and one sees; one descends and one sees no longer,
but one has seen.
There is an art of conducting oneself . . .
by the memory of what one saw higher up.
When one no longer sees, one can at least still know.
— René Daumal

Sometimes the catalyst is curiosity, and sometimes it is despair.
— Michael Lee

If I learned anything about mountains while I was hiking the Long Trail, it was this: What goes up will always go down and then back up again. Peaceful plateaus are few and far between. I also learned to be appreciative of all of it. When I was going up, I hoped for a little down. When I was going down, my body was relieved by a little up. When I walked across a plateau, I could take in the view of the ups and downs that lay behind me and wonder about the ones that waited ahead.

I found the best way to deal with the pendulum swings of the transformative process was to ground myself in good old fashioned creative labor. In those times when I began to feel the swing begin in either direction, I turned toward those activities that anchored me in the present moment through my body.

In addition to breath, meditation and Yoga postures, I found centered ground in many other ways. Getting out onto the earth, into the vastness of nature, was one. The hiking that started it all remains a favorite method of regaining perspective. I also like wrapping my fingers around my knitting needles or my paint brushes. I lavish attention on my pets and grandchildren, dig in my gardens, and make big pots of soup on the woodstove. Even quietly dusting shelves or sweeping floors connect me to the middle place of the pendulum's arc.

What I have learned from pendulums is to ride the ups *and* the downs by examining and letting go of my attachments to both.

CONCLUSION

It's also helpful to realize that this body that we have,
that's sitting right here right now . . . with its aches and pains . . .
is exactly what we need to be fully human, fully awake, fully alive.
— Pema Chödrön

Each night of Long Trail hiking found me at a simple hut or lean-to cooking dinner and remembering the day's adventures in my journal. Sometimes it was difficult to put the chain of experience into words. It feels this way now as I attempt to summarize my point of view. My body is full of a multitude of sensation, emotions and thoughts as I untangle what I wish to say in closing.

As I transcribed, from my journal, the details of personal experience for this text, I re-experienced them in my body. When I wrote about the Long Trail, my shoulder and upper back tightened up. Writing about my car accident engaged my left body, who said, "Oh, I remember that! It felt like this!" As I wrote about my youth, I felt as if I were coming down with a cold – my body re-visiting the childhood ailments associated with my abuse. None of these body remembrances lasted for long, nor were they as severe as they originally were. Recognizing what was happening and why, I was able to thank them, and they softened away. They were actually wonderfully timed affirmations of what I have been attempting to write about.

In untangling the knots in my body and then weaving together the loose ends of their colorful treads, I am discovering the fabric of who I am. The more embodied I become – the more I *am* my body – the better I understand myself and the world around me. A doorway to self; my body guides me toward ever-expanding knowledge. As the door opens, more is revealed, and new edges and questions evolve.

The postures of life never end, and I am grateful they continue. This means I get to be alive! For, as Chödrön says above, being alive provides me with the incredible opportunities to be both fully human and fully awake to the sensations of abiding wisdom (consciousness). The everyday miracle of my body tells me this is so.

My dear friend Debra Lubar created and plays the elder character Rose in a memorable stage production of Jewish wisdom. Rose offers this: "The truth? What is it? It is a satchel, what contains everything you can imagine and everything you cannot – all mingled together with the good, the bad and the miracles." I find, in order to maintain a consistent openness to my embodied flow of life information, I need to remain the beginner. I do not know it all. Waking up each day with the open mind of a beginner creates healthy internal transformative space. I need to remind myself to let go of blockages, to be loose to life, to be curious rather than resistant and to allow the spontaneous stuff of discovery occur. I am hosting the continual tea party.

Inviting Others

I teach Yoga classes several times per week in addition to my own practice. I offer many of the perspectives of this text to my students. It is inspiring when I learn they are beginning to discover ways to come to their own bodies for guidance and knowledge. Such was the case with L, a dedicated student of the body and Yoga. She agreed to share her moving account of how she came to understand something important about herself through body awareness.

>   *For months I had been plagued with a reoccurring pain near my bottom left rib. The pain would appear suddenly and it made it difficult to get a full breath of air into my lungs. It was a sharp pain. Each time the pain would appear, it would stay for 3-5 days.*
>
>   *I sought help from my chiropractor, who recommended strengthening my core muscles more, which I was trying to achieve through various activities. I continued all of my physical activities mostly, except when the 'rib thing' would start in on me, and then*

I would take it easy, do what I could. And so this pain went on and off for some time.

One of my favorite activities included Yoga. In the beginning of Yoga, I had purely taken it for the physical benefits. I had always been a physical person and not very emotional. I had always believed pain had a reason – a reason such as a wrong movement or overdoing it, etc. I never much thought about my pain being caused by emotions or from stress. I went through the motions in each Yoga class, always physically and never mentally. What I didn't realize is slowly I was absorbing bit s and pieces of phrases that my instructor was telling the class. I pretty much thought it never applied to me. The Yoga continued and the rib pain came and went over and over again.

A phrase was starting to hang around in my head a lot and it was my instructor's phrase. It said something about 'when you have a reoccurring pain you might think about what is really going on in your life. No matter how foreign this phrase was at first, it was starting to come around more frequently. I was still persistent in thinking that my pain was there because of something I had done physically.

I don't exactly remember the moment I figured it out, but it all seemed so simple once I made the discovery. The discovery was my rib would start to hurt whenever our sixteen-year-old son and I had a disagreement or if I had been excessively worrying about him. It seems so obvious how could I not have noticed? Once I accepted what was going on in my life the rib pain ceased and has not come back to me.

I believe my mind was desperately trying to tell my body, 'Hey! We are a unit – together!' I didn't like the confrontations with my son because I hated the feelings it brought up and I would try to ignore those feelings. But since my brain wouldn't acknowledge those feelings, my body had to take the pain. A sharp pain in the rib (one that takes your breath away) will make anyone pay attention after a while – some longer than others.

Another interesting note about the rib ordeal is while talking to my instructor about this over a period of a couple of months, she asked if I'd ever experienced anything like the rib pain before. I remembered that when I was pregnant with my son I had some discomfort and stiffness in this same region.

I have learned so much from my rib pain. It has taken me almost forty years to realize you must acknowledge your feelings because if you do not your feelings will come knocking on your door in the form of pain, disease or addiction. I now see so many people who seem to always be in pain from one thing or another and it makes me wonder, 'What's going on in there?' I also know it's something each person has to experience and discover for themselves."

Questioning Being

In her poem, *The Turtle*, Mary Oliver writes:

The turtle breaks from the blue-black skin of the water, dragging her shell with its mossy scutes across the shallows and through the rushes and over the mudflats, to the uprise, to the yellow sand, to dig with her ungainly feet a nest, and hunker there spewing her white eggs down into the darkness, and you think of her patience, her fortitude, her determination to complete what she was born to do – and then you realize a greater thing – she doesn't consider what she was born to do. She's only filled with an old blind wish. It isn't even hers but came to her in the rain or the soft wind, which is a gate through which her life keeps walking. She can't see herself apart from the rest of the world or the world from what she must do every spring, crawling up the high hill, luminous under the sand that has packed against her skin. She doesn't dream, she knows she is a part of the pond she lives in, the tall trees are her children, the birds that swim above her are tied to her by an unbreakable string.

I often wonder just how advanced humans really are. Why is it that we question our being – our existence? "Who am I? Why am I?" Does our ability to question life and self put us at the top of the ladder of species, or at the bottom?

I don't suppose the butternut tree outside my window contemplates consciousness. It seems to easily know how to be in the world. I'll bet it doesn't fret about the future or spend hours unraveling its past. The black cat, snoozing on the end of my bed, hasn't the time to consider the meaning of his life. I'm quite sure he already knows. I'm also quite sure, as he opens a clear eye in my direction, that he is amused with the amount of work I am attempting to do. One look in the eye of the bobcat that crossed my headlights a few nights ago, or the gray wolf I encountered in Yellowstone Park this summer, was enough to instantly inform me they knew much more than I. The barred owl, whose preserved wing now fans out across one wall of my study, died from flying into our van. He did not seem to regret his short and simple life – yet he clung fiercely to the love for it at the end.

I think, perhaps, we're at the bottom after all. But hey, there's no way to go but up!

Cellular Changes – Backward, Sideways and Forward

My mother, Barbara, passed from this life in July 2004. It always seemed as though she was afraid of everything from thunderstorms to speaking her own mind. At times, when she observed the stubborn outspokenness of my adolescence, I think she was even afraid of me. What she wasn't openly afraid of, she managed to worry about. So, it was with a certain amount of caution that I approached her doorstep in 1996 with the odd news that I was about to spend twenty-three or more days in the wilderness alone.

I awaited her response. She looked at me with her usual worried eyes. She held her breath. "Is this something you really *want* to do?"

"Yes"

(Pause.) "Aren't you afraid?"

"No."

(Pause.) "Good for you!" she concluded.

That was it? To my surprise, the conversation casually turned to particulars about the trip and normal family stuff. She never attempted to talk me out of it, nor did she act the least bit worried. In fact, she almost seemed excited.

On the day I 'finished' the Long Trail, I called my daughters and my sisters to tell them I was out of the woods. They all reacted with general acceptance of my feat, their lives too busy to pay long attention to what crazy Mom/Elissa had been up to.

As I mentioned earlier, I was struggling with my attachment to recognition and self-validation at this time. At the edge of this struggle, hurting from head to toe, I stopped over to see Mom. All along, I had operated under the assumption that Mom would be the least apt to get it – to understand why I had done this hike. On many levels, I still didn't comprehend my own reasons. With the exception of Dave's enthusiastic support, this had so far been a lonely endeavor. I had no reason to believe that Mom would be anything but simply glad I had not broken any body parts or lost too much weight. But my assumptions were unfounded, as they often are.

I learned Dave had provided Mom with a large map of the state of Vermont, which she had enshrined on her kitchen table. Framed by the background of her red and white, checkered tablecloth, the big green map looked alive with the energy she had been pouring into it and, consequently, into me.

Each night before going to bed, she had highlighted with a magic marker the length of trail I had likely covered that particular day. Every night she had taken pride in my steps as if they were her own. Every night she prayed that I would get to the border safely. Not only did Mom 'get it', she had, in her own way, hiked along with me every step of the way. She had been an intentional, large part of the universal presence I felt as I walked.

That day, when I looked into her eyes, they were different. They were brighter, younger, clearer, unworried and less tired. When she showed me her map project, her smile told me I was not the only one who had changed through this experience. On a deep, cellular, genetic level, Mom had changed, too. And I sensed she knew it, although she did not or could not express it.

My mother's eyes, actions and approaches to life following this event became further evidence that shifts in awareness occur in a collective manner. She was more self-confident, calm and accepting of things than she had been before. This state lasted until she was unable to keep caring for herself and to forget who I was. When she died, I was with her. She bravely rode out on a thunderstorm, the likes of which once frightened her.

So now I wonder, how far backwards in my genetic lineage do my shifts in awareness go? Do they cross the parallels of existence and shift the DNA in my resting grandmothers and great-grandmothers? Do they reach forward into the seed bodies of my grandchildren's children? Certainly, I can see how my changes move sideways into my daughters and granddaughters. They are the present evidence that growth in one is growth in all. And I have yet to realize how these children are also changing me, one cell at a time.

Close on the heels of these questions and insights comes responsibility. Knowing transformation has a value larger than we can imagine, we must continue to do the work of awareness, to say "yes" to change and to remember why.

The body — the process of embodiment — is an essential element of a transformative practice. Life's information rests within the body's cells and tissues waiting for us to notice. Coming to one's body with respectful inquiry can gradually lead to knowledge of one's authenticity. Through the body, one comes home to self.

EPILOGUE

"Mornin' Rob," I spoke across the counter while peering down into my bag for breakfast funds.

"Mornin'," he replied while simultaneously making change for the person in front of me. I swear this Bristol Bakery icon can multitask better than most moms of small children. "Hey, this has been a great group of people this time! We've really enjoyed getting to know them! It's been nice that some have been here long enough to get to know their names. When will they be back?"

Rob was referring to the large group of Phoenix Rising Yoga Therapy students who had been in Bristol, Vermont – some of them for twenty days – participating in our professional training program. They had become beloved regular customers, sometimes ending up there more than once a day, hungry and eager to connect with the locals. They had descended on the town from all over the globe – Japan, Iceland, Australia and, of course, the United States.

In September of 2006, I was blessed with the opportunity to form a partnership with my dearest mentor and teacher, Karen Hasskarl, to lease the creative rights, responsibilities and international training center of Phoenix Rising Yoga Therapy from its creator, Michael Lee. Several roads converged to make this possible: Michael was ready to move on to exciting new discoveries and ideas. The building that had housed the training center in West Stockbridge, Massachusetts was being sold. Karen was imagining a move back to Vermont, where she had always been the happiest, but she also wanted to continue with Phoenix Rising Yoga Therapy, expanding her current role as Director of Programs. And I found myself in the right place at the right time.

I had become the director of the Phoenix Rising Yoga Teacher and Group Facilitator programs, and was staffing some of the other Yoga Therapy trainings as well. And, I already lived in Vermont! So the plan easily evolved to move Phoenix Rising to Vermont with Karen and I at the helm.

Within a week of the decision to do so, we had found a space in a to-be-renovated, perfectly located facility in my hometown, the place where my adventures in self-discovery had all begun. We moved Phoenix Rising Yoga Therapy in November 2006, hosting our first training there the following January.

Two years before this move, when I had finished writing the first draft of this book, I felt done with the lessons and pain of the 1996 fitness center loss that plunged me into depression and the first steps of that Long Trail hike. In spite of the embarrassment and degradation I created for myself, I had remained in the community that I felt I had "let down" by my shortcomings. I eventually allowed myself to be buoyed-up by the loving support of a town which chose to continue to respect and include me rather than dwell on the details of my "failure," even when it had affected many other lives.

But, until this day in the Bakery, I was not yet fully aware that there was one last piece of that old event left undone.

When I looked up from digging around in my purse and saw the genuine appreciation in Rob's smile, a deep connecting warmth spread from my chest out to each limb, and up and down my spine. Something broke free in my heart – some last bit of holding back. It was as if the last piece of a puzzle plunked squarely into place, the completion of something important, a big exhale, a welcomed opening.

Walking back to the training center, I realized that in the past few years I had harbored a niggling of guilt at letting down my community. Through my willingness to stay with myself and grow from my experience, however, I had somehow stepped into a do-over. I had brought a community-sustaining business home with me as I had found "home" within me. Rob's words sealed the completion of this particular adventure in self-healing. I felt like I could finally breathe!

Later that day the training program ended, and Karen and I said "Goodbye" to Rob's students with the usual hugs, tears and well-wishes. The training center quiet once again, I plunked down at my computer to catch up on a few e-mails. As I typed my right shoulder began to talk with an angry tone, vying for my immediate attention. After some internal argument, I turned off the computer and smiled to myself. Just when I thought I was done . . .

BIBLIOGRAPHY

Agnes, Michael. (Ed.). (2003). *Webster's New World dictionary: Fourth Edition.* New York. Pocket Books.

Ajaya, Swami. (1983). *Psychotherapy East and West: A Unifying Paradigm.* Honesdale, PA. Himalayan International Institute of Yoga Science and Philosophy of the USA.

Al Huang, Chungliang & Lynch, Jerry. (1995). *Mentoring: The TAO of Giving and Receiving Wisdom.* San Francisco. HarperCollins.

Anderson, Sherry Ruth &Hopkins, Patricia. (1991). *The Feminine Face of God: The Unfolding of the Sacred.* New York. Bantam Books.

Baldwin, E., Longhurst, B., McCracken, S., Ogborn, M., & Smith, G. (1999). *Introducing Cultural Studies.* Athens, GA. The University of Georgia Press.

Bankart, Peter. (1997). *Talking Cures: A History of Western and Eastern Psychotherapies.* Pacific Grove, CA. Brooks Cole Publishing Co.

Benson, Herbert. (1996) *Timeless Healing: The Power and Biology of Belief.* New York. Simon & Schuster.

Blum, Ralph. (1982). *The Book of Runes.* New York. St. Martin's Press.

Bouanchaud, Bernard. (1997). *The Essence of Yoga: Reflections on the Yoga Sutras of Patañjali.* Portland, OR. Rudra Press.

Charet, Francis. (1-16-03). *Body, Mind and Synchronicity: A Talk at Goddard College Spring Residency.* Plainfield, VT. Goddard College.

Chödrön, Pema. (2001). *The Places That Scare You: A Guide to Fearlessness in Difficult Times.* Boston. Shambhala Publications, Inc.

Collins, Peter E. (1976). *Wilhelm Reich: A Synthesis of His Work and Mind.* Goddard College. BA Senior Study.

Cope, Stephen. (1999). *Yoga and the Quest for the True Self.* New York. Bantam Books.

Cope, Stephen. (5-14-03). *Self-soothing and the Transformation of Narcissism: Talk, Workshop and Panel Discussion.* Lenox, MA. Psychotherapy & Spirituality Conference. Kripalu Center for Yoga and Health.

Coster, Geraldine. (1972). *Yoga and Western Psychotherapy.* New York. Harper & Row, Publishers.

Dychtwald, Ken. (1977). *Bodymind.* New York. Jeremy P. Tarcher/Putnam.

Epstein, Mark. (1995). *Thoughts Without a Thinker: Psychotherapy from a Buddhist Perspective.* New York. Basic Books.

Farhi, Donna. (1996). *The Breathing Book: Good Health and Vitality Through Essential Breath Work.* New York. Henry Holt & Co.

Feldenkrais, Moshe. (1977). *Awareness through Movement: Health Exercises for Personal Growth.* New York. Harper & Row, Publishers.

Feldenkrais, Moshe. (1985). *The Potent Self: A Guide to Spontaneity.* San Francisco. Harper & Row, Publishers.

Feuerstein, Georg. (1998). *Tantra: The Path of Ecstasy.* Boston. Shambhala Press.

Feuerstein, Georg. (2000). *The Shambhala Encyclopedia of Yoga.* Boston. Shambhala Publications, Inc.

Feuerstein, Georg. (2001). *The Yoga Tradition: Its History, Literature, Philosophy and Practice.* Prescott, Arizona. Holm Press.

Ford, Clyde. (5-16-03). *The Healing of Persons, The Healing of Nations, Embodied Wisdom in Embattled Times: Talk, Workshop and Panel Discussion.* Lenox, MA. Psychotherapy & Spirituality Conference. Kripalu Center for Yoga and Health.

Friedman, Lenore (ED) & Moon, Susan (ED). (1997). *Being Bodies: Buddhist Women on the Paradox of Embodiment.* Boston. Shambhala Publications, Inc.

Gates, Rolf & Kenison, Katrina. (2002). *Meditations from the Mat: Daily Reflections on the Path of Yoga.* New York. Anchor Books.

Gavin, James. (1988). *Bodymoves: The Psychology of Exercise.* Harrisburg, PA. Stackpole Books.

Gendlin, Eugene T. (1981) *Focusing*. Toronto. Bantam Books.

Goldstein, Kurt. (1939) *The Organism: A Holistic Approach to Biology Derived from Pathological Data in Man*. Boston. Beacon Press.

Goleman, Dan. (5-17-03). *Overcoming Destructive Emotions: How Meditation Changes the Brain*. Lenox, MA. Psychotherapy & Spirituality Conference. Kripalu Center for Yoga and Health.

Grand, Ian J. (1992). *Of Tissue States and Thermostats: Clinical Observations*. (Spring/Summer) The Journal of Somatic Experience. Vol. 4. No. 2. Human Sciences Press.

Grof, Stanislav. (1998). *The Cosmic Game: Explorations of the Frontiers of Human Consciousness (Series in Transpersonal and Humanistic Psychology*. Albany, New York. State University of NY Press.

Grof, Stanislav (ED) & Grof, Christina (ED). (1989). *Spiritual Emergency: When Personal Transformation Becomes a Crisis*. New York. Jeremy P. Tarcher/ Putnam Books.

Grof, Stanislav & Grof, Christina. (1992). *The Stormy Search for the Self: A Guide to Personal Growth Through Transformational Crisis*. New York. Putnam Publishing Group.

Gurman, Alan S. & Messer, Stanley B. (1995). *Essential Psychotherapies: Theory & Practice*. New York, Guilford Press.

Harris, Judith. (2001). *Jung and Yoga: The Psyche-Body Connection*. Toronto. Inner City Books.

Harvey, Andrew. (2000). *A Journey in Ladakh: Encounters With Buddhism*. Boston. Houghton Mifflin Co.

Harvey, Andrew. (1991). *Hidden Journey: A Spiritual Awakening*. New York. Henry Holt and Company.

Jacobs, Hans. (1961). *Western psychotherapy and Hindu Sadhana: A Contribution to Comparative Studies in Psychology and Metaphysics*. London. George Allen & Unwin, LTD.

Johanson, Greg & Kurtz, Ron. (1991). *Grace Unfolding: Psychotherapy in the Spirit of the Tao-te Ching*. New York. Bell Tower.

Johnson, Robert A. (1991). *Owning Your Own Shadow: Understanding the Dark Side of the Psyche*. San Francisco. HarperSanFrancisco.

Judith, Anodea. (1996). *Eastern Body, Western Mind: Psychology and the Chakra System as a Path to the Self*. Berkeley, CA. Celestial Arts.

Kegan, Robert. (1989). *The Evolving Self: Problem and Process in Human Development*. Cambridge, MA. Harvard University Press.

Keller, Doug. (2001). *Refining the Breath: Pranayama in the Anusara Style of Yoga*. Riding, VA. DoYoga Productions.

Kornfield, Jack. (2000). *After the Ecstasy, The Laundry: How the Heart grows Wise on the Spiritual Path*. New York. Bantam Books.

Kurtz, Ron. (1988). *Body Centered Psychotherapy: The Hakomi Method*. Ashland, Oregon. The Hakomi Institute.

Kurtz, Ron & Prestera, Hector. (1976). *The Body Reveals: An Illustrated Guide to the Psychology of the Body*. New York. Harper & Row.

Ladinsky, Daniel. (1996). *I Heard God Laughing: Renderings of Hafiz*. Walnut Creek, CA. Sufism Revisited.

Ladinsky, Daniel, Translator. (2003). *The Subject Tonight is Love: Sixty Wild and Sweet Poems of Hafiz*. USA. Penguin Books.

Lakoff, G. & Johnson, M. (1999). *Philosophy in the Flesh: The Embodied Mind and Its Challenge to Western Thought*. New York. Basic Books.

Lawliss, Frank G. (1996). *Transpersonal Medicine: A New Approach to Healing Body-Mind-Spirit*. Boston. Shambhala Publications, Inc.

Lee, Michael. (1997). *Phoenix Rising Yoga Therapy: A Bridge from Body to Soul*. Deerfield Beach, Florida. Health Communications, Inc.

Levine, Stephen. (1979). *A Gradual Awakening*. New York. Anchor Books.

Lowen, Alexander. (1958). *The Language of the Body*. New York. Collier Books.

Marieb, Elaine N. (2000). *Essentials of Human Anatomy & Physiology*. San Francisco. Addison Wesley Longman, Inc.

Mehta, S., Mehta, M. & Mehta, S. (2001). *Yoga the Iyengar Way: The New Definitive Illustrated Guide*. New York. Alfred A Knopf.

Mindell, Arnold. (1977). *Dreambody: The Body's Role in Revealing the Self*. Portland, Oregon. Lao Tse Press.

Moore, Thomas. (5-17-03). *Psychotherapy as Care for the Soul: Talk, Workshop and Panel Discussion*. Lenox, MA. Psychotherapy & Spirituality Conference. Kripalu Center for Yoga and Health.

Murphy, Michael. (1992). *The Future of the Body: Explorations Into the Further Evolution of Human Nature*. New York. Jeramy P. Tarcher/Putnam.

Myss, Caroline. (1996). *Anatomy of the Spirit: The Seven Stages of Power and Healing*. New York. Three Rivers Press.

Oliver, Mary. (1992). *New & Selected Poems*. Boston. Beacon Press.

Pearsall, Paul. (1998). *The Heart's Code: The New Findings About Cellular Memories and Their Role in the Mind/Body/Spirit Connection*. New York. Broadway Books.

Pelletier, Kenneth R. (1977). *Mind as Healer, Mind as Slayer: A Holistic approach to Preventing Stress Disorders*. New York. Dell Publishing Company.

Pert, Candace B. (1997). *Molecules of Emotion: The Science Behind Mind-Body Medicine*. New York. Touchstone.

Perls, Frederick, Hefferline, Ralph F. & Goodman, Paul. (1951). *Gestalt Therapy: Excitement and Growth in the Human Personality*. New York. Julian Press.

Pierrakos, Eva. (1990). *The Pathwork of Self-transformation*. New York. Bantam Books.

Plumb, Sylvia (EDT). (1996). *The Green Mountain Club Long Trail Guide: Vermont Hiking Trails Series*. Waterbury, Vermont. Green Mountain Club.

Pringer, Byron Christopher. (1995). *Fascial-Based Emotional Memory Storage System*. Retreived August 11, 2003 from http:/members.aol.com/bridge22/FasciaMemTheory. html.

Ramachandran. (1999). *Phantoms in the Brain*. New York. William Morrow and Co.

Rama, Swami, Ballentine, Rudolph & Ajaya, Swami. (1976). *Yoga and Psychotherapy: The Evolution of Consciousness*. Honesdale, PA. The Himalayan Institute of Yoga Science and Philosophy.

Ram Das. (1971). *Be Here Now*. New York. Crown Publishing Group.

Ravrindra, Ravi. (1984). *Whispers From the Other Shore: A Spiritual Search – East and West*. Wheaton, Illinois. Quest Books.

Rham, Cat de & Gill, Michèle. (2001). *The Spirit of Yoga*. London. Thorsons.

Rodegast, Pat & Stanton, Judith. (1985). *Emmanuel's Book: A Manual for Living Comfortably in the Cosmos*. New York. Bantam Books.

Rogers, Carl R. (1961). *On Becoming a Person: A Distinguished Psychologist's Guide to Personal Growth and Creativity*. Boston. Houghton Mifflin Company.

Rossi, Ernest L. (1986). *The Psychobiology of Mind-Body Healing: New Concepts of Therapeutic Hypnosis*. New York/London. W.W. Norton Company, Inc.

Roth, Sheldon. (1990). *Psychotherapy: The Art of Wooing Nature*. Northvale, NJ. Jason Aronson, Inc.

Satchidananda, Sri Swami. (1988). *The Living Gita: The Complete Bhagavad Gita*. Yogaville, VA. Integral Yoga Publications.

Satprem. (Mahak, Francine & Venet, Luc, Translators). (1982). *The Mind of Cells or Willed Mutation of the Species*. New York. Institute for Evolutionary Research.

Scaravelli, Vanda. (1991). *Awakening the Spine: the Stress-Free New Yoga that Works with the Body to Restore Health, Vitality and Energy*. New York. Harper Collins Publishers.

Schwartz, Richard C. (5-15-03). *The Internal Family Systems Model: Releasing the Self in Psychotherapy – Talk, Workshop & Panel Discussion*. Lenox, MA. Psychotherapy & Spirituality Conference. Kripalu Center for Yoga and Health.

Scientists Discover 'Second Brain' in the Stomach (Filed November 3, 2000). Retrieved September 9, 2003 from http://www.ananova.com/news/story/sm_105441.html.

Selye, Hans. (1956) *The Stress of Life*. New York. McGraw Hill Book Company.

Shanker, Uday. (1992) *Psycho-Analysis VS Psychosynthesis or Yoga: A Comparative Study of Psychoanalysis and Yoga Psychology*. New Delhi. Enkay Publishers Pvt. Ltd.

Shapiro, Debbie. (1990) *The Bodymind Workbook: Exploring How the Mind and the Body Work Together*. Shaftsbury, Dorset. Element Books, Limited.

Sheldrake, Rupert. (1987) *Mind, memory, and Archetypal Morphic Resonance and the Collective Unconscious*. Retrieved September 10, 2003 from Sheldrake Online. http://www.sheldrake.org/papers/morphic/morphic1_paper.html.

Simonton, O. Carl. (1987) *Getting Well: A Step-by-Step Guide to Overcoming Cancer for Patients and Their Families*. New York. St. Martin's Press. Audio Renaissance Tapes, Inc.

Small, Jacquelyn. (May 16, 2003). *Soul-Based Psychologies: Gift to Addiction Recovery and Other Human Plights – Talk, Workshop & Panel Discussion*. Lenox, MA. Psychotherapy & Spirituality Conference. Kripalu Center for Yoga and Health.

Sri Aurobindo. (1948) *The Synthesis of Yoga*. Pondicherry, India. Sri Aurobindo Ashram Press.

Stiles, Mukunda. (2000) *Structural Yoga Therapy: Adapting to the Individual*. York Beach, Maine. Samuel Weiser, Inc.

Taylor, Kylea. (1995) *The Ethics of Caring: Honoring the Web of Life in Our Professional Healing Relationships*. Santa Cruz, CA. Hanford Mead Publishers.

Temoshok, Lydia. (1992) *The Type C Connection: The Behavioral Links to Cancer and Your Health*. New York. Random House.

Tolle, Eckhart. (1999) *The Power of Now: A Guide to Spiritual Enlightenment*. Novato, CA. New World Library.

Tulku, Tarthang. (1977) *Time, Space, and Knowledge: A New Vision of Reality.* Berkeley, CA. Dharma Publishing.

Underwood, Anne. (May 7, 2001) *Religion and the Brain: How We're Wired for Spirituality.* Newsweek. New York. Newsweek, Inc.

Von Franz, Marie-Louise (1996) *The Interpretation of Fairy Tales.* Boston. Shambhala Publications.

Vrinte, Joseph. (1995, b. 1949) *The Concept of Personality in Sri Aurobindo's Integral Yoga Psychology and A. Maslow's Humanistic/Transpersonal Psychology.* New Delhi. Munshiram Manoharlal Publishers, Pvt. Ltd.

Wilber, Ken. (2000) *Integral psychology: Consciousness, Spirit, Psychology, Therapy.* Boston & London. Shambhala Press.

Willis, Claire & Marvin, Carolyn. (May 15, 2003) *Creating a Container for Transformation: Talk, Workshop and Panel Discussion.* Lenox, MA. Psychotherapy & Spirituality Conference. Kripalu Center for Yoga and Health.

Wolf, Kate. Another Sundown Publishing Co. (recorded 1993) Music and Lyrics of *Across the Great Divide.* Recorded by Nanci Griffith. *Other Voices/ Other Rooms.* Nashville. Elextra Entertainment.

ABOUT THE AUTHOR

Elissa Cobb is the Program Director of Phoenix Rising Yoga Therapy located in Bristol, Vermont. She has more than twenty years of combined practice and teaching experience in fitness/health consulting, body/mind and movement practices, Yoga and Yoga Therapy. Elissa now leads Phoenix Rising training programs worldwide and is an active speaker at mind/body industry conferences and symposia. *The Forgotten Body* is her first book.

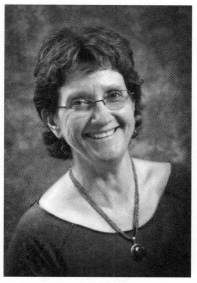

Loveworks Photographic, Bristol, VT